AF364245

Experimental Approaches to Biopharmaceutics and Pharmacokinetics

Experimental Approaches to Biopharmaceutics and Pharmacokinetics

Dr. Suresh Bandari
M.Pharm, Ph.D
Professor & Principal

Vijay Kumar Nagabandi
M.Pharm., Ph.D
Assistant Professor

Dr. Jukanti Raju
M.Pharm., Ph.D
Former Associate Professor

St. Peter's Institute of Pharmaceutical Sciences
Hanamkonda, Warangal.

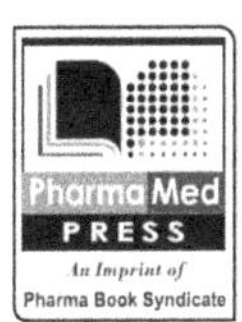

PharmaMed Press
An imprint of Pharma Book Syndicate

A Unit of BSP Books Pvt. Ltd.
4-4-309/316, Giriraj Lane,
Sultan Bazar, Hyderabad - 500 095.

Published by

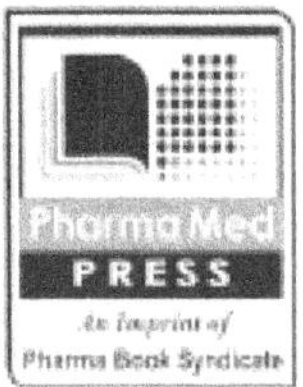

PharmaMed Press

An imprint of Pharma Book Syndicate

A Unit of BSP Books Pvt. Ltd.
4-4-309/316, Giriraj Lane, Sultan Bazar, Hyderabad - 500 095.
Phone: 040-23445600, 23445688; Fax: 91+40-23445611
E-mail: info@pharmamedpress.com
www.pharmamedpress.com/pharmamedpress.net

ISBN: 978-93-89974-74-4

PREFACE

The first edition of "Experimental Approaches to Biopharmaceutics and Pharmacokinetics" will cater the basic experimental aspects of Biopharmaceutics and Pharmacokinetics.

This book is an comprehensive resource for design of experiments in disintegration, dissolution, diffusion, protein binding studies, factors affecting drug release, drug interactions, methods to enhance drug dissolution, kinetic modeling of drug release, bioavailability studies, bioequivalence studies, creatinine clearance, nomograms, statistical analysis such as t-test and ANOVA, pharmacokinetics of single dose and multiple doses as per one compartment modeling and two compartment modeling, non compartment kinetics, non linear kinetics and viva voce questions.

This invaluable text differs from other practical manuals on fundamental principles of biopharmaceutics and pharmacokinetics, as it has both experimental and relevant theoretical aspects in the form of appendices.

CONTENTS

EXPERIMENT 10

EXPERIMENT 11

EXPERIMENT 12

EXPERIMENT 13

EXPERIMENT 14

EXPERIMENT 15

EXPERIMENT 16

EXPERIMENT 17

EXPERIMENT 18

EXPERIMENT 19

APPENDIX 7

APPENDIX 8

APPENDIX 9

APPENDIX 10

EXPERIMENT 1

CALIBRATION CURVE OF SALICYLIC ACID BY COLORIMETRY

AIM

To construct a calibration curve of salicylic acid using colorimetric method.

CHEMICALS

Salicylic acid, Hydrochloric acid (1%v/v), Ferric chloride, Distilled water.

PRINCIPLE

The increasing concentrations of salicylic acid is treated with 1% ferric chloride reagent (1g $FeCl_3$ in 100 mL of 1% Hydrochloric acid). The free phenolic hydroxyl group present in salicylic acid reacts with the reagent and forms a violet coloured complex i.e., ferric salicylate which is proportional to the concentration of salicylic acid.

PROCEDURE

Ferric chloride reagent is prepared by adding 1 gm of $FeCl_3$ to 100 mL of 1% HCl (1mL concentrated hydrochloric acid added to 100mL of distilled water).

Stock solution of salicylic acid (1mg/mL) is prepared by dissolving 100 mg of salicylic acid in few mL of methanol and made up to 100 mL with distilled water in a volumetric flask. 10 mL of this stock solution is diluted with 100 mL distilled water to get 100 µg/mL salicylic acid solution.

Take the respective samples in each test tube, add the reagent and distilled water to make total volume of 10 mL (as per mentioned in table) and measure the absorbance of the violet colored complex using

UV-Visible spectrophotometer at wavelength of 525 nm against blank sample (without salicylic acid).

Volume of stock solution (mL)	Volume of reagent (mL)	Distilled water to make 10 mL	Concentration of Salicylic acid (μg/mL)	Absorbance
0 (Blank)	1	9	0	0
1	1	8	10	--
2	1	7	20	--
3	1	6	30	--
4	1	5	40	--
5	1	4	50	--
6	1	3	60	--

Plot a graph taking concentration on X-axis and observed absorbance values on Y-axis, draw a best fit line and record r^2 value (regression coefficient) and equation of straight line.

REPORT

Calibration Curve of salicylic acid is plotted and the concentration of unknown sample can be determined from interpolation of calibration curve.

CALIBRATION CURVE OF DICLOFENAC SODIUM BY UV SPECTROPHOTOMETRY

AIM

To construct a calibration curve of diclofenac sodium using UV spectrophotometric method.

CHEMICALS

Diclofenac sodium, Disodium hydrogen phosphate, Sodium hydroxide, Potassium dihydrogen phosphate, Distilled water.

PRINCIPLE

The absorbance increases linearly with increase in the concentration of diclofenac sodium. Record the absorbance values at 276 nm and plot a graph taking concentration (independent variable) on X-axis and absorbance (dependent variable) on Y-axis and draw a best fit line.

PROCEDURE

Preparation of working stocks of Diclofenac sodium

100 mg dissolved in100 mL of 6.8 pH phosphate buffer (1mg/mL)

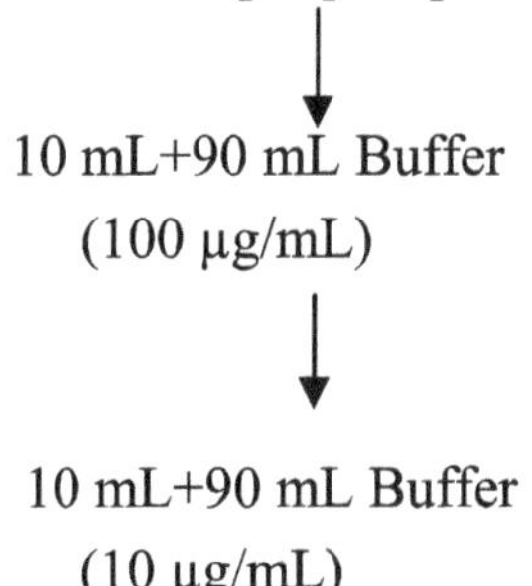

Take the respective sample in each test tube, and phosphate buffer to make total volume of 10 mL (as per mentioned in table) and measure the absorbance of the solution using UV-Visible spectrophotometer at wavelength of 276 nm against blank.

Stock solution	Volume of stock solution (mL)	Buffer required to make 10mL	Conc. of diclofenac sodium (µg/mL)	Absorbance
0 µg/mL	0 (Blank)	10	0	0
10 µg/mL	2	8	2	--
10 µg/mL	4	6	4	--
10 µg/mL	6	4	6	--
10 µg/mL	8	2	8	--
100 µg/mL	1	9	10	--
100 µg/mL	1.2	8.8	12	--
100 µg/mL	1.4	8.6	14	--

Plot a graph taking concentration on X-axis and observed absorbance values on Y-axis, draw a best fit line and record r^2 value (regression coefficient) and equation of straight line.

REPORT

Standard graph of diclofenac sodium is plotted and the concentration of unknown sample can be determined from interpolation of calibration curve.

EXPERIMENT 3

LINEAR REGRESSION AND CORRELATION COEFFICIENT

AIM

To derive a straight line equation by least squares procedure and measure the linear relationship of the variables.

THEORY

Straight lines are found in many theoretical relationships in physical and biological chemistry. First order and zero order kinetics can be expressed in a linear form. Michaelis-menton's equation for enzyme kinetics and Arrhenius relationship used in stability studies can be transformed into linear forms. The reasons for the desirability of straight line relationships include the ease of extrapolation and interpolation as well as simplification of the determination of the parameters of the line, the slope and the intercept.

One of the problems in estimating the slope and intercept from practical data is the variability and the plot does not clearly define a straight line. In pharmacokinetic study, the X variable (time) can be measured with great accuracy. The dependent variable (concentration), is variable due to biologic system, analytical error, human error etc. The practical data can be fit into a line, using the straight line equation.

Correlation is a measure of the linear relationship between two variables. The correlation coefficient (r^2) is calculated to know whether a linear relationship really exists between the two variables or not. If X and Y are variables,

$$\text{Correlation coefficient } (r^2) = \frac{\Sigma\, xy - (\Sigma x \times \Sigma y)/n}{\sqrt{\Sigma\left(x - \overline{x}\right)^2 \Sigma\left(y - \overline{y}\right)^2}}$$

The correlation coefficient can vary between +1 and -1. A correlation coefficient of +1 would result if all points fall exactly on a single line with positive slope, this is a perfect positive correlation and vice versa.

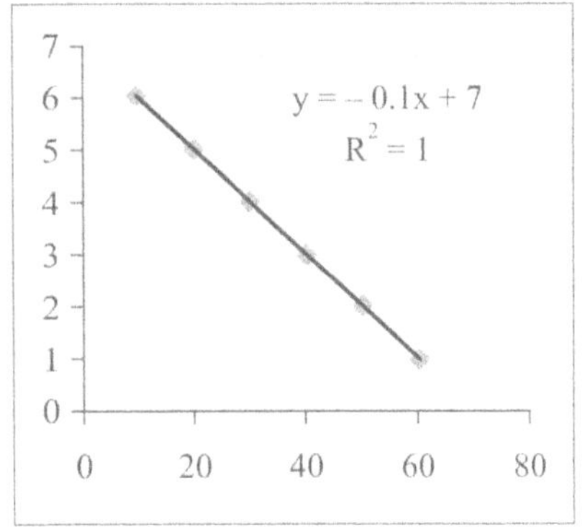

<table>
<tr><td>Perfect correlation
with (– ve) slope</td><td>Perfect correlation
with (+ ve) slope</td></tr>
</table>

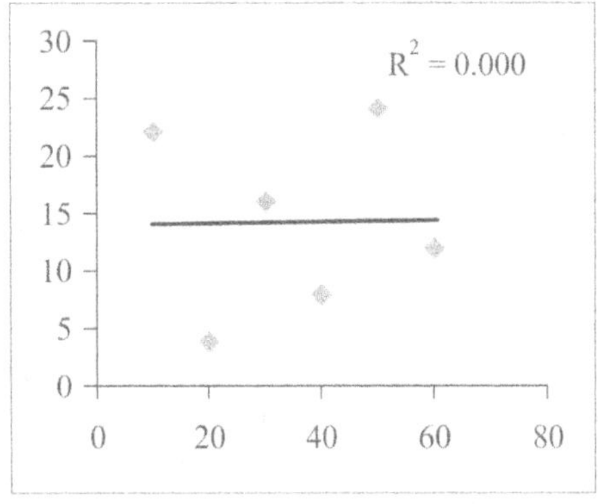

No Correlation

PROCEDURE

Data: The reaction rate of a drug was measured at different temperatures. The following data were obtained. Using linear regression of the data, find out the parameters governing the straight line relationship and comment on the linearity of the variables.

Temperature, X (^{o}C)	10	20	30	40
Reaction rate, Y (mg/hr)	0.241	0.492	0.710	0.978

Solution

Calculate and set up the following table

x (Temp)	y (Reac. Rate)	$x - \bar{x}$	$y - \bar{y}$	$\left(x - \bar{x}\right)\left(y - \bar{y}\right)$	$\left(x - \bar{x}\right)^2$
10	0.241	− 15	− 0.364	5.464	225
20	0.492	− 5	− 0.113	0.566	25
30	0.710	5	0.105	0.524	25
40	0.978	15	0.373	5.591	225

$$\bar{x} = 25 \quad \bar{y} = 0.6053 \quad \Sigma\left(x - \bar{x}\right)\left(y - \bar{y}\right) = 12.145 \quad \Sigma\left(x - \bar{x}\right)^2 = 500$$

$$\text{Slope} = \frac{\Sigma\left(x - \bar{x}\right)\left(y - \bar{y}\right)}{\Sigma\left(x - \bar{x}\right)^2}$$

$$= 12.145 / 500 = 0.0243$$

$$y = mx + c$$

$$\text{Intercept} = C = \bar{y} - m\bar{x}$$

$$C = 0.6053 - 0.0243 \times 25 = -0.002$$

Therefore the equation of the straight line describing the variables is

$$Y = 0.0243\ X - 0.002$$

Correlation coefficient

x (temp)	y (Reac. Rate)	xy	$x - \bar{x}$	$\left(x - \bar{x}\right)^2$	$y - \bar{y}$	$(y - \bar{y})^2$
10	0.241	2.41	-15	225	-0.364	0.133
20	0.492	9.84	-5	25	-0.113	0.013
30	0.710	21.3	5	25	0.105	0.011
40	0.978	39.12	15	225	0.373	0.139

$$\bar{x} = 25 \quad \bar{y} = 0.6053 \quad \Sigma\, xy = 72.67 \quad \Sigma\, xy = 500 \quad \Sigma\left(y - \bar{y}\right)^2 = 0.2954$$

$$\Sigma\, x = 100 \quad \Sigma\, y = 2.421$$

$$r = \frac{\Sigma\, xy - (\Sigma x \times \Sigma y)/n}{\sqrt{\Sigma\left(x - \bar{x}\right)^2\, \Sigma\left(y - \bar{y}\right)^2}} = \frac{72.67 - 242.1/4}{\sqrt{500 \times 0.2954}} = \frac{12.14}{12.15} = 0.9991$$

REPORT

The data points are linear since the correlation coefficient value is nearer to 1.

EXPERIMENT 4

DISINTEGRATION OF TABLETS

AIM

To determine the disintegration time of given tablets.

PROCEDURE

Uncoated/ Film coated/ Sugar coated tablets

Take 6 units of Uncoated/ Film coated/ Sugar coated tablets and place in the six tubes of disintegration apparatus. The apparatus is operated using distilled water or 0.1 N HCL maintained at $37 \pm 2^\circ$C as the immersion fluid for specified time (15 min for uncoated, 30 min for film coated and 60 min for sugar coated). Remove the assembly from the liquid at the end of the test. Determine whether the tablets are disintegrated completely within the specified limits as per pharmacopoeia. If one or two tablets fail to disintegrate, repeat the test on 12 additional tablets; not less than 16 of the total 18 tablets tested must disintegrate in specified time.

Enteric coated tablets (I.P)

Take 6 units of enteric coated tablets and place in the six tubes of disintegration apparatus. The apparatus is operated (without disc) using simulated gastric fluid or 0.1N HCL maintained at $37 \pm 2^\circ$C as the immersion fluid. After 2 hours of operation, lift the basket from the fluid and observe the tablets. The tablets do not show any evidence of disintegration, cracking or softening. Replace the immersion fluid and continue the process (with disc) for one hour by immersing the baskets in simulated intestinal fluid or mixed phosphate buffer pH 6.8 maintained at $37 \pm 2^\circ$C as the immersion fluid. Record the time taken for the tablets to disintegrate completely at the end of the test.

Check Appendix 2 for further details

REPORT

The average DT is calculated for uncoated and coated tablets and the test passes if it meets the requirements as per I.P.

EXPERIMENT 5

DISSOLUTION OF CONVENTIONAL TABLETS

AIM

To perform the dissolution (*in vitro* drug release studies) of Conventional (uncoated) tablets.

PROCEDURE

1. Place the stated volume of dissolution medium about 900 mL in the dissolution apparatus as specified in the individual monograph.

2. Set the temperature of the medium to $37°C \pm 0.5°C$ and also set the RPM specified in the monograph.

3. Place six tablets in each vessel individually and immediately start the apparatus.

4. At predetermined time intervals, withdraw an aliquot (5 mL) of sample from the zone midway between surface of the dissolution medium and the top of the rotating blade, not less than 1cm from the vessel walls and replace with equal volume of fresh medium. Filter the sample by passing through 0.45 μm filter.

   Note: Care should be taken that the temperature of replacement medium should be maintained at $37°C \pm 0.5°C$

5. Dilute the samples suitably with dissolution medium and record the absorbance of the samples at its λmax and determine the concentration of drug in the sample from the standard plot.

6. By using the time and concentration data of the samples, calculate the percent drug release (Refer Appendix 3; Table No: 2)

7. Plot a graph, taking time on X-axis and % drug release on Y-axis and calculate dissolution parameters like dissolution efficiency, mean dissolution time etc.

REPORT

Dissolution study of given dosage form was performed and the results obtained are given in the following table.

Tablet	% Drug release	Dissolution Efficiency	Mean Dissolution time

EXPERIMENT 6

DISSOLUTION OF ENTERIC COATED TABLETS

AIM

To perform the dissolution profile (*In vitro* drug release studies) of enteric coated tablets.

PRINCIPLE

1. Enteric-coated tablets (Gastric-resistant tablets) are tablets covered with one or more layers of coatings intended to resist the gastric fluid but to release their active ingredient(s) in the intestinal fluid. For this purpose, substances such as cellulose acetate phthalate and anionic copolymers of methacrylic acid and its ethers are used for providing tablets with a gastric-resistant coating.

2. Coated tablets have a smooth, usually polished and often colored, surface; a broken section examined under a lens shows a core surrounded by one or more continuous layers of a different texture.

METHODS FOR TESTING ENTERIC COATED TABLETS

1. *Method A*

The apparatus type to be used for testing a particular drug product is specified in the drug monograph. The product is first tested in 0.1N HCl for 2 hours, and then changed to pH 6.8 by adding 0.2M tribasic sodium phosphate. Final adjustment of the pH of the dissolution medium can be made either with 2N NaOH or 1 N HCl if necessary. The test is then generally carried for 45 min. Specifications are set in the individual drug monographs.

2. *Method B*

Dissolution is carried out in the apparatus specified in the individual drug monograph. This method involves testing the drug product in 0.1N HCl for 2 hours, and then draining the acidic medium and replacing it with a pH 6.8 mixed phosphate buffer medium.

PROCEDURE

1. Place the stated volume of dissolution medium pH 1.2 (0.1N HCl) about 900 mL in the dissolution apparatus specified in the individual monograph.

2. Set the temperature of the medium to 37°C ± 0.5°C and also set the RPM specified in the monograph.

3. Take six tablets and place each unit in each vessel and immediately start the apparatus.

4. At predetermined time interval, withdraw an aliquot (5 mL) of sample from the zone midway between surface of the dissolution medium and the top of the rotating blade, not less than 1cm from the vessel walls and replace with equal volume of fresh medium.

5. After 2hours of sampling, adjust/change the pH of the dissolution medium to 6.8 as per the procedure described above.

6. Repeat the sampling at predetermined time intervals and replace with equal volume of dissolution medium.

   Note: care should be taken that the temperature of replacement medium should be maintained at 37°C ± 0.5°C

7. Record the absorbance of the samples and determine the concentration of drug in the sample from the calibration curve.

8. By using the time and concentration data of the samples, calculate the percent drug release (Refer appendix 3; Table no 2)

9. Plot a graph, taking time on X-axis and cumulative % released on Y-axis and calculate dissolution efficiency

ACCEPTANCE CRITERIA (USP)

The test passes, if the enteric coated tablets meet the following acceptance criteria mentioned in table

Stage 1: *Acidic medium (0.1N HCl)*

Level	No of tablets tested	Acceptance Criteria
A1	6	No individual unit exceeds 10% dissolved
A2	6	Avg of 12 units (A1+A2) is not more than 10% dissolved and no individual unit is greater than 15% dissolved
A3	12	Avg of 24 units (A1+A2+A3) is not more than 10% dissolved and no individual unit is greater than 25% dissolved

Stage 2: *Basic medium (6.8 pH buffer)*

Level	No of tablets tested	Acceptance Criteria
S1	6	Each unit is not less than Q* + 5%
S2	6	Avg of 12 units (S1+S2) is equal to or greater than Q, and no unit is less than Q-15%
S3	12	Avg of 24 units (S1+S2+S3) is equal to or greater than Q, not more than 2 units are less than Q-15% and no unit is less than Q-25%

Note: *Q* is the amount of dissolved active ingredient specified in the individual monograph, expressed as % of the stated amount.*

REPORT

Dissolution study of given dosage form was performed and the results obtained are given in the following table

Tablet	% Drug release		Dissolution Efficiency
	Acidic media	Basic Media	

EXPERIMENT 7

DISSOLUTION OF SUSTAINED RELEASE (SR) TABLETS

AIM

To perform the dissolution study (*In vitro* drug release studies) of sustained release tablets.

THEORY

Sustained release dosage form is a continuously releasing medication over an extended period of time after administration of a single dose (these dosage forms generally follows first order release profile). Whereas, controlled drug delivery system is the one which delivers the drug at a predetermined rate for a specified period of time (these dosage forms generally follows zero order release profile).

Advantages

1. Frequency of drug administration is reduced.

2. Patient compliance can be improved.

3. Blood level oscillations can be reduced because a more even blood level is maintained.

4. Total amount of the dose administered can be reduced.

Disadvantages

1. Termination of therapy is not possible.

2. Less flexibility in adjusting dosage regimens.

3. Designed for normal population, consequently, disease states that alter drug disposition, significant patient variation, and so forth are not accommodated.

Comparisons between sustained release and controlled release

Sustained Release Dosage form	Controlled Release Dosage form
Release the drug slowly over a prolonged period of time	Release the drug at predetermined rate over a prolonged period of time
It depends on concentration of drug in formulation	It is independent of concentration of drug in formulation
It follows first order kinetics	It follows zero order kinetics
Ex: Voveran SR	EX: OROS osmotically control system

Characteristics of drugs unsuitable for SR dosage forms

Not effectively absorbed in the lower intestine - Riboflavine, Ferrous salts

Absorbed and excreted rapidly (half-life<1hr) - Penicillin G, Furosemide

Long biological half-lives (>12hr)   - Diazepam, Phenytoin

Large doses required (>1g)   - Sulphonamides

Drugs with low Therapeutic Index   - Phenobarbital, Digoxin

No clear advantage for SR formulation   - Griseofulvin (poor sol)

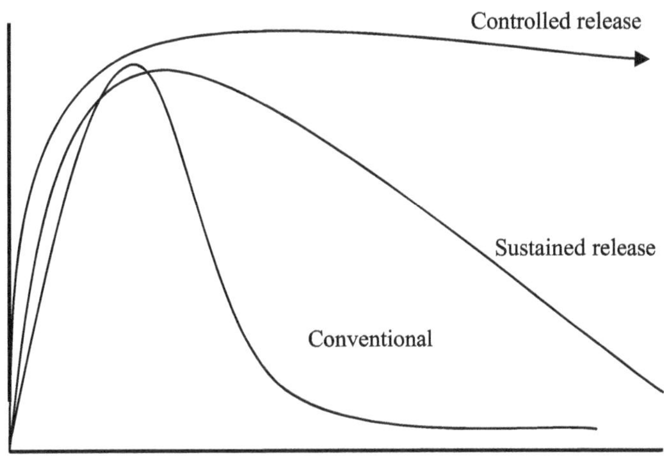

Fig. 1 Typical release profiles for Conventional, Sustained release and Controlled release dosage forms.

PROCEDURE

1. Place the stated volume of dissolution medium about 900 mL in the dissolution apparatus specified in the individual monograph.

2. Set the temperature of the medium to 37°C ± 0.5°C and also set the RPM specified in the monograph.

3. Take six SR tablets and place each SR tablet individually in each vessel and immediately start the apparatus.

4. At predetermined time intervals, withdraw an aliquot (5 mL) of sample from the zone midway between surface of the dissolution medium and the top of the rotating blade, not less than 1cm from the vessel walls and replace with equal volume of fresh medium. Filter the sample by passing through 0.45 μm filter.

    Note: care should be taken that the temperature of replacement medium should be maintained at 37°C ± 0.5°C.

5. Record the absorbance of the samples and determine the concentration of drug in the sample from the standard plot.

6. By using the time and concentration data of the samples, calculate the percent drug release. (Refer appendix 3, table No: 2)

7. Plot a graph taking time on X-axis and cumulative % released on Y-axis and calculate dissolution efficiency.

8. Plot zero order, first order, higuchi plot, korsemeyer peppas plot, and hixson crowell plots and determine the order and mechanism of drug release from the graphs.

    Note: See Appendix 5 for details.

Acceptance Criteria: The drug release from SR products is assessed at three levels (given in below table). The first point would be set at a testing period corresponding to a dissolved amount of 20 per cent to 30 per cent. The second point would be set at around 50 per cent release. The final point would ensure almost complete release that is generally understood as more than 80 per cent release. Carry out the test for the test-times indicated on the label of the product.

Level	Time point (h)	% Drug Released
L1	1	30
L2	4	50
L3	8	80

Note: Time points and corresponding % drug released values varies from product to product as per individual monographs

REPORT

Tablet	% of Drug Release	R^2 value				
		Zero order	First Order	Higuchi	Korsmeyer	Hixson-Crowell

EXPERIMENT 8

DISSOLUTION STUDY OF DIFFERENT DOSAGE FORMS

AIM

To conduct and compare the dissolution profile of different dosage forms of given drug (Cephalexin).

REQUIREMENTS

Potassium dihydrogen phosphate, Sodium hydroxide, Three different dosage forms of any drug (tablets, capsule, suspension), Distilled water, Test tubes, pH meter, Volumetric flasks, Dissolution test apparatus (Type-I & II), Pipettes.

PRINCIPLE

- ➢ Dissolution (absorption) for different dosage forms decreases in the following order:

  Solutions > Emulsions > Suspensions > Capsules > Tablets > Coated tablets > Enteric coated tablets > Sustained release dosage forms.

- ➢ In solutions drug is in solubilized form and has the fast absorption as the major rate limiting step, dissolution is absent.

- ➢ In emulsions & suspensions the particles diffuse from the dosage form into solution. The major rate-limiting step in the absorption of the suspension is the dissolution.

- ➢ In capsules the gelatin shell has to disintegrate and then drug release takes place.

- ➢ The tablets have to undergo disintegration, deaggregation and then dissolution, which is relatively a slow process.

PROCEDURE

1. Place 900 ml of the phosphate buffer solution in each vessel of the dissolution apparatus.

2. Assemble the apparatus and equilibrate the medium to $37 \pm 0.5°C$. USP paddle type is used for all dosage forms and for capsules use sinkers.

3. Now place the formulation in each vessel and operate the apparatus with 50 rpm.

4. Withdraw 5 ml of the sample for every predetermined interval from the zone midway between surface of the dissolution medium and the top of the rotating blade, not less than 1cm from the vessel walls.

5. Replace the aliquots withdrawn for analysis with equal volumes of fresh dissolution medium.

   Note: care should be taken that the temperature of replacement medium should be maintained at $37°C \pm 0.5°C$.

6. The samples are collected in clean and dry test tubes.

7. The absorbance of the drug in each sample is measured using UV-Visible spectrophotometer at λ_{max}. Dilutions are made if required.

8. Percentage release of the drug is calculated at each time interval using the A (1 %, 1cm) or slope of the standard graph. Check the individual monograph in pharmacopoeia for A (1 %, 1cm).

   If A (1%, 1cm) is used, Slope = (Absorbance×10,000)/(A (1%,1cm)

9. Dissolution efficiency is calculated from the graph between percent of drug release vs. time. Data obtained with each dosage form are compared. (Refer Appendix 3; Table No: 2)

REPORT

Dissolution efficiency of each dosage form is calculated and reported

Dosage form	% Drug Release	Dissolution Efficiency	Mean Dissolution Time
Tablets			
Capsules			
Suspension			

EFFECT OF POLYMORPHISM ON DRUG DISSOLUTION

AIM

To conduct and compare the dissolution profile (*In vitro* drug release studies) of various polymorphic forms of given drug (Salicylic acid).

REQUIREMENTS

Beakers, Glass rods, Test tubes, Ice cubes, Conical flasks, Funnels, Volumetric flasks, Solvents (Acetone, Methanol, Ethanol, Chloroform and Water) and drug.

PRINCIPLE

Depending upon the internal structure, a solid can exist either in a crystalline or amorphous form. When a substance exists in more than one crystalline form, the different forms are designated as **Polymorphs** and the phenomenon as **Polymorphism.**

Polymorphs are of two types:

- Enantiotropic polymorph is the one which can be reversibly changed into another form by altering the temperature or pressure e.g. sulfur, and

- Monotropic polymorph is the one which is completely stable at all temperatures and pressures e.g. glyceryl stearates.

The polymorphs differ from each other with respect to their physical properties such as solubility, melting point, density, hardness and compression characteristics. They can be prepared by crystallizing the drug from different solvents under diverse conditions. The existence of the polymorphs can be determined by using techniques such as optical crystallography, X ray diffraction, differential scanning calorimetry, etc.

The order for dissolution of different solid forms of drug is Amorphous> Metastable Polymorph> Stable Polymorph

PROCEDURE

1. Preparation of various polymorphs of given drug:

(a) Dissolve the drug in different solvents separately like Acetone, Methanol, Ethanol and Chloroform, Acetone + Methanol, and Chloroform + Ethanol or any other solvents in different ratios.

(b) The dissolved drug is re crystallized by transferring the above solution to ice water.

(c) Filter the each solvent, collect the crystals and air dried.

(d) Then the obtained crystals are observed under microscope for determining shape and size of the crystals and to determine the polymorphism

(e) Then determine the melting point of each crystalline form

2. Dissolution Studies of obtained Polymorphs:

1. Place 100 mg of drug in dissolution vessel and add 900 ml of distilled water to vessel.

2. Assemble the apparatus and operate the apparatus with 50 rpm after achieving $37\pm 0.5^{\circ}C$

3. Withdraw 5 ml of the sample for every predetermined time interval from the zone midway between surface of the dissolution medium and the top of the rotating blade, not less than 1cm from the vessel walls.

4. Replace the aliquots withdrawn for analysis with equal volumes of fresh dissolution medium.

5. Collect the samples in clean and dry test tubes.

   Note: care should be taken that the temperature of replacement medium should be maintained at $37^{\circ}C \pm 0.5^{\circ}C$.

6. Dilute suitably and measure the absorbance of the drug in each sample using UV-Visible spectrophotometer at λ_{max}.

7. Calculate percentage release of the drug at each time interval using the standard graph. Calculate dissolution efficiency from the graph between percent of drug release vs. time. (Refer Appendix 3; Table No: 2).

8. Repeat the same experiment for all crystals obtained in the same way and compare the result obtained.

9. Calculate the dissolution efficiency and mean dissolution time of each crystalline form and report them.

REPORT

The dissolution efficiency and mean dissolution time of each crystal was calculated and reported.

Polymorph	Size & Shape	Melting Point	Dissolution Efficiency	Mean Dissolution Time

EXPERIMENT 10

EFFECT OF COMPLEXATION ON SOLUBILITY AND DISSOLUTION RATE

AIM

To determine the effect of complexation on solubility and dissolution rate of a given drug

REQUIREMENTS

Beakers, funnels, conical flasks, mechanical shaker, dissolution apparatus, β-Cyclodextrin, distilled water, acetone, and drug

PRINCIPLE

Complexation is one of several ways to favorably enhance the physico chemical properties of pharmaceutical compounds. It can be defined as the reversible association of substrate and ligand to form a new species. Various complexes formed can be differentiated as molecular complexes, metal complexes, inclusion complexes and ion exchange compounds.

Cyclodextrins (CDs) are classic examples of compounds that form inclusion complexes. These complexes are formed when a ''guest'' molecule is partially or fully included inside a ''host'' molecule e.g., CD with no covalent bonding. When inclusion complexes are formed, the physicochemical parameters of the guest molecule are disguised or altered.

CD formulations provide improved aqueous solubility to poorly soluble drugs, and the drug: CD complex often exhibits improved dissolution characteristics compared to other formulations of the drug. These two features can provide for an improvement in oral bioavailability when solubility and the rate of dissolution are limiting the availability of the drug for absorption.

Basically, complexes are pharmacologically inert and must dissociate either at the absorption site or following absorption in to the systemic circulation. Several examples where complexation has been used to enhance the drug bioavailability are:

1. Enhanced dissolution through formation of soluble complex e.g. ergotamine tartarate-caffeine complex and hydroquinone – digoxin complex,

2. Enhanced lipophilicity for better membrane permeability e.g. caffeine – PABA complex, and

3. Enhanced membrane permeability e.g. enhanced GI absorption of heparin (normally not absorbed from the GIT) in presence of EDTA which chelates calcium and magnesium ions of the membrane.

Complexation can be deleterious to drug absorption due to formation of poorly soluble or poorly absorbable complex e.g. complexation of tetracycline with divalent and trivalent cations like calcium (milk, antacids), iron (hematinics), magnesium (antacids) and aluminium (antacids). Reasons for poor bioavailability of some complexes are failure to dissociate at the absorption site and large molecular size of the complex that cannot diffuse through the cell membrane-for example, drug-protein complex.

PROCEDURE

Step 1: Preparation of Cyclodextrin-Drug complex (solid dispersion)

Solid dispersions are prepared by solvent evaporation method.

1. An appropriate amount of cyclodextrin is added to solution of drug in 15 mL of ethanol.

2. The solution is stirred at 60 rpm and the solvent is evaporated under reduced pressure at 40°C in a rotary flash evaporator for 2 h.

3. The obtained solid dispersions are subsequently stored in a vacuum oven at room temperature for 48 h to remove the residual solvent.

4. The dried solid residue is pulverized and sieved through 250 μm sieve. The samples obtained are stored in desiccator until further analysis.

Step 2: Determination of solubility of the pure drug and drug-cyclodextrin complex

1. Take 5ml of water into previously dried 2 glass vials. Add excess amount of drug and drug complex into the vials separately.

2. Then keep them for agitation on a rotary shaker for 24 h/until equilibrium is achieved.

3. After 24 hrs/after attaining equilibration remove the vials from the shaker.

4. The samples are filtered using membrane filter.

5. The filtered samples are assayed spectrophotometrically at its specified λ_{max} and solubility of drug and complex are obtained.

Step 3: Determination of dissolution rate of the pure drug & drug-cyclodextrin complex

(a) Place 900 ml of the distilled in each vessel of the dissolution apparatus.

(b) Assemble the apparatus and equilibrate the medium to $37\pm0.5°C$.

(c) Now place the 100 mg of pure drug powder in each vessel. Operate the apparatus with 50 rpm.

(d) Withdraw 5 ml of the sample for every predetermined time interval from the zone midway between surface of the dissolution medium and the top of the rotating blade, not less than 1cm from the vessel walls.

(e) Replace the aliquots withdrawn for analysis with equal volumes of fresh dissolution medium.

   Note: care should be taken that the temperature of replacement medium should be maintained at $37°C \pm 0.5°C$.

(f) The samples are collected in clean and dry test tubes.

(g) The absorbance of the drug in each sample is measured using UV-Visible spectrophotometer at λ_{max}. Dilutions are made if required.

(h) Percentage release of the drug is calculated at each time interval using the standard graph. (Refer Appendix 3 Table No 2).

(i) Repeat the same experiment with drug-cyclodextrin complex by taking weight equivalent to 100 mg of pure drug.

REPORT

The solubility and dissolution rate of pure drug and drug-cyclodextrin complex are calculated and compared.

EXPERIMENT 11

COMPARATIVE DISSOLUTION STUDIES OF MARKETED PRODUCTS AND TREATMENT OF DATA BY USING ANOVA

AIM

To conduct the comparative dissolution studies of various brands of given drug (same dosage form) and treatment of data by **ANOVA**

REQUIREMENTS

Tablets (6 different brands & 6 tablets for each brand), Distilled water, Test tubes, volumetric flasks, and Dissolution test apparatus (Type-II)

PROCEDURE

1. Place 900 ml of the distilled water in each vessel of the dissolution apparatus.

2. Assemble the apparatus and equilibrate the medium to $37 \pm 0.5°C$.

3. Now place the first formulation in each basket. Operate the apparatus at 100 rpm.

4. Withdraw 5 ml of the sample for every predetermined time interval from the zone midway between surface of the dissolution medium and the top of the rotating blade, not less than 1cm from the vessel walls.

5. Replace the aliquots withdrawn for analysis with equal volumes of fresh dissolution medium.

6. Collect the samples in clean and dry test tubes.

7. Dilute suitably and measure the absorbance of the drug in each sample using UV-Visible spectrophotometer at λ_{max} of the drug.

8. Calculate percent drug release at each time interval using the standard graph. Calculate dissolution efficiency from the graph between percent drug release vs. time. Data obtained with each tablet are compared.

9. Repeat the same experiment with all other 5 brands.

10. Analyze the data obtained by applying Multiple ANOVA (Refer Appendix 6)

REPORT

Dissolution studies of six different brands were performed and data obtained was treated with multiple ANOVA. It was found that all the brands are found equivalent (or) not equivalent.

IN VITRO DRUG DIFFUSION FROM OINTMENT BASES

AIM

To assess *in vitro* drug diffusion from various ointment bases.

CHEMICALS

Cholesterol, stearyl alcohol, white beeswax, white soft paraffin, propylene glycol, sodium lauryl sulphate, polyethyleneglycol-400, polyethyleneglycol-4000, Agar-Agar, salicylic acid, ferric chloride and hydrochloric acid.

PRINCIPLE

Ointments are semisolid preparations for external application to the body. Ointments are used primarily as protectives, vehicles or bases for the topical application of medicinal substances. Ideally, an ointment base should be compatible with the skin, stable, smooth, non-irritating, non-sensitizing, inert and able to release its incorporated medication. Based on composition ointment bases can be classified into four types as follows:

1. *Oleaginous ointment base*

These are also referred as hydrocarbon bases. They contain fixed oils of vegetable origin, fat and semisolid hydrocarbons obtained from petroleum. The disadvantages of these bases are their water absorbing capacity is low and they have a tendency to become rancid. They are excellent emollients.

2. *Absorbent ointment base*

Absorbent ointment bases are also referred as emulsifiable bases. The term 'Absorbent' is used here to denote the water absorbing property of these bases. Generally they are anhydrous substances which have the property of absorbing considerable quantity of water and still retaining their consistency. No water is used in basic formula.

3. *Emulsion ointment base*

Emulsion ointment bases are actually semisolid emulsions. They are also called as water removable bases. They are of two types o/w and w/o these both bases will permit the incorporation of some additional amount of water without reducing consistency below that of a soft cream. o/w can be removed readily from skin whereas w/o emulsions are better emollients and protectants.

4. *Water soluble ointment base*

These are also termed as water washable ointment bases. They are prepared from higher ethylene glycol polymers. The polymers have a high range of molecular weights. The polymers are non-volatile, water soluble and unctuous. They do not hydrolyze or deteriorate and will not support mold growth. They also find application in preparation of suppositories.

PROCEDURE

Prepare 2% Agar-Agar medium (dissolve 2g in 100mL of distilled water and heat it to get clear solution) and pour 30mL into each petri plate and allow it to solidify. Then make three cups of same diameter with the help of a borer.

1. *Oleaginous or Hydrocarbon or Simple ointment base*

White wax	-	0.5 g
White petrolatum	-	9.5 g
Salicylic acid	-	0.2 g

Melt white wax in suitable dish by heating on water bath and add white petrolatum warm until it liquefies, then dissolve the salicylic acid. Discard the heat and stir the mixture until it begins to congeal.

2. *Absorption ointment base or Hydrophilic ointment base (USP)*

Cholesterol	-	0.3 g
Stearyl/Cetyl alcohol	-	0.3 g
White bees wax	-	0.8 g
White petrolatum	-	8.6 g
Salicylic acid	-	0.2 g

Melt stearyl alcohol and white wax on water bath. Then add cholesterol and white petrolatum stir until it completely dissolves. Add salicylic acid and remove from water bath and stir until the mixture congeals.

3.   *Emulsion or Water removable ointment base*

Stearyl/Cetyl alcohol	-	2.5 g
White petrolatum	-	2.5 g
Propylene glycol	-	1.2 g
Sodium lauryl sulphate (SLS)	-	0.1 g
Distilled water	-	3.7 mL
Salicylic acid	-	0.2 g

Melt stearyl alcohol and white petrolatum on water bath and dissolve salicylic acid in it. In another container take 3.7mL of distilled water, add propylene glycol and SLS and warm it to 75°C. Add aqueous portion into oil portion and stir continuously until it congeals.

4.   *Water washable or Water soluble ointment base*

Polyethylene glycol 4000	-	4 g
Polyethylene glycol 400	-	6 g
Salicylic acid	-	0.2 g

Melt PEG-4000 on water bath and add PEG-400 and mix it uniformly. Then dissolve salicylic acid. Discontinue heating and stir it continuously until it congeals.

Fill equal quantity of ointment in the cups made in agar plate (triplicate) and keep aside for 4 hours. Then pour 1% ferric chloride reagent on the surface of agar plate and observe the violet colour spread around the cavity. Measure the diameter of color zone around the cup. Calculate the average diameter for each ointment base.

REPORT

The drug diffusion from various ointment bases is in the following descending order.

EXPERIMENT 13

IN VITRO DRUG PERMEATION (DIFFUSION) STUDY OF OINTMENT

AIM

To conduct the permeation study of marketed ointment by using franz diffusion cell.

REQUIREMENTS

Diffusion Medium (Based on drug), Sampling cannula, 5ml syringe, diffusion cell (Franz), polymeric membrane (gelatin sheet/dialysis membrane) and ointment (marketed).

PRINCIPLE

Ointments are homogeneous, semi solid preparations intended for external application to the skin or certain mucous membranes for emollient, protective, therapeutic or prophylactic purposes where a degree of occlusion is desired. They usually consist of solutions or dispersions of one or more medicaments in suitable bases. Ointments may contain suitable auxiliary substances such as antioxidants, stabilizers, thickeners and emulsifiers and, when the base might support the growth of microbial contaminants, suitable antimicrobial preservatives. Drug release pattern from the any of the dosage form is to be determined as one of the evaluation parameter for the *in vitro - in vivo* correlation. If the dosage form is orally administered like tablet or capsule or suspension, by simply conducting *in vitro* dissolution test one can correlate the *in vivo* bioavailability. But in case of topically administered dosage forms like ointments, creams and gels etc., it is not feasible to conduct the dissolution test for determination of drug release pattern as this test will not correlate in vivo bioavailability. For these kinds of dosage forms it is possible to determine the drug release pattern by conducting diffusion studies. With the diffusion cell it is possible to study various diffusion processes in ointments, gels and the penetration of active agents through the membrane (gelatin sheet/dialysis membrane/any animal membrane to conduct *ex vivo* studies) into the receptor medium, wherein its concentration may be determined.

PROCEDURE

1. Take one diffusion (Franz) cell which has two compartments (Donor and Receptor) with a sampling provision in lower (receptor) compartment.

2. Place magnetic bead in the lower compartment and fill with suitable diffusion medium up to the maximum level.

3. Sandwich the membrane between two compartments of the diffusion cell such that it should be always in contact with diffusion medium in the receptor compartment.

4. No solution is added to the upper compartment.

5. Weigh accurately 1g of ointment or quantity equivalent to 1 dose, spread evenly on to the membrane and place the diffusion cell on magnetic stirrer.

6. Start the magnetic stirrer after adjusting the temperature to 37°C at 100 rpm.

7. Take 1 ml of sample from the lower compartment using the cannula at predetermined time intervals and replace with fresh medium.

8. Measure the absorbance of the sample and calculate the concentration of drug diffused using standard graph and calculate permeability coefficient and flux of the drug through the membrane. (Refer appendix 4 for details)

REPORT

Permeability coefficient and flux of drug in a given ointment was calculated and reported.

EXPERIMENT 14

PROTEIN BINDING STUDIES

AIM

To determine the effect of protein (albumin) binding on the diffusion of drug through the membrane.

REQUIREMENTS

Potassium dihydrogen phosphate, Sodium hydroxide, Diffusion cell, Egg albumin powder, gelatin sheet/dialysis membrane, syringe with sampling cannula and drug

PRINCIPLE

A drug in the body can interact with several tissue components of which the two major categories are blood and extravascular tissues. The interacting molecules are generally macromolecules such as proteins, DNA or adipose. The phenomena of complex formation with protein are called as protein binding of drugs. The protein bounded drug is both pharmacodynamically and pharmacokinetically inert. A bound drug is also restricted since it remains confined to a particular tissue for which it has greater affinity. Moreover, such a bound drug, because of its enormous size, cannot undergo membrane transport and thus its half life is increased.

Binding of drugs falls into 2 classes

1. Binding of drugs to blood components like plasma proteins, blood cells, etc..,

2. Binding of drugs to extra vascular proteins, fats, bones, etc.

Plasma Protein-drug binding

Once the drug is available in systemic circulation, it may interact with components of blood such as plasma proteins, blood cells, and hemoglobin. The main interaction of drug in the blood compartment is with the plasma proteins which are present in abundant amounts and in

33

large variety. The binding of drugs to plasma proteins is reversible. The extent of binding of drugs to various plasma proteins is:

Albumin > α1-acid glycoprotein > lipoproteins > globulins

The methods to study kinetics of protein binding and to determine stoichiometric ratio are

1. Equilibrium dialysis
2. Dynamic dialysis
3. Ultrafiltration

Binding sites and Binding constants can be determined by plotting the data obtained using the following

(a)   Direct plot method
(b)   Double Reciprocal plot
(c)   Scatchard plot

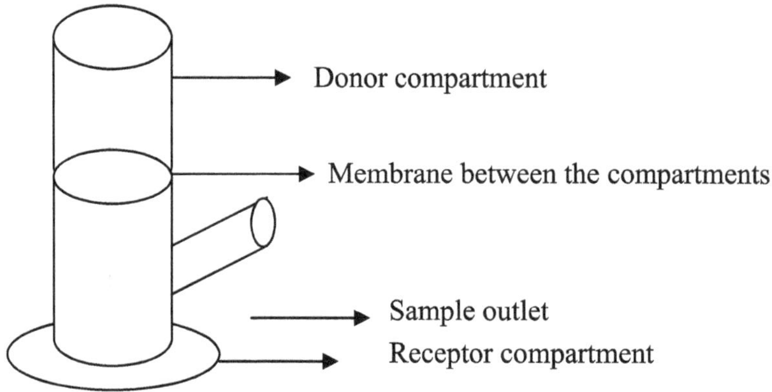

Franz Diffusion cell

In the present experiment effect of concentration of proteins (egg albumin) on drug binding is studied. As the concentration of protein increased, free drug concentration available for diffusion will decrease. That means more the protein content more will be the binding. After attaining drug binding saturation level further increase in protein level will not affect the protein binding

PROCEDURE

1. Prepare 1 mg/ml solution of drug in 7.4 pH Buffer

2. Prepare 1 mg/ml solution of protein (egg albumin powder) in 7.4 pH Buffer

3. Fill the lower chamber (receptor) of diffusion cell with the 7.4 pH buffer

4. Sandwich the membrane between two compartments of the diffusion cell such that it should be always in contact with diffusion medium in the receptor compartment.

5. Assemble the apparatus and place the diffusion cell on magnetic stirrer.

6. Add 2 ml of drug solution and 1 ml of protein solution to the upper chamber (donor chamber) of the diffusion cell from the top. (Drug: Protein -1: 0.5 ratio)

7. Fill the volume of the donor compartment with 7.4 pH buffer to maintain constant level for all trials.

8. Run the magnetic stirrer at 100 rpm for 6 h.

9. Withdraw the samples from receptor compartment at predetermined time intervals and analyze the sample for drug content.

10. Calculate the % drug diffused and calculate permeability coefficient and flux of the drug through the membrane.

11. Repeat the same experiment with 1:1 (2 ml drug solution + 2ml protein solution) and 1:2 (2 ml drug solution + 4 ml protein solution)

12. Repeat the same experiment for pure drug (control) without protein solution (2 ml of drug solution only).

REPORT

Protein binding study was conducted by diffusion method at different ratios of protein, and it was found that the flux and permeability coefficient of the drug was in the following order.

EXPERIMENT 15

IN VITRO DRUG – DRUG INTERACTION STUDIES

AIM

To determine the *in vitro* drug-drug interaction by using UV spectrophotometer.

THEORY

When the pharmacological activity of one drug is altered by the concomitant use of another drug, is known as drug-drug interaction.

Pharmacodynamic interactions are those in which the activity of the drug at its site of action is altered by another drug.

1. Potentiation

2. Synergism

3. Antagonism

Pharmacokinetic interactions

Some drugs may affect Absorption, Distribution, Metabolism, and Excretion of one drug by others.

Object drug	Precipitant drug	Influence on Object drug
Tetracycline	Antacids, food and Ca ions	Unabsorbable complexes
Sulphonamides, Aspirin	Antacids	Enhanced absorption rate
Anticoagulants	Phenylbutazone, Salicylates	Increased clotting time
Oral contraceptives	Barbiturates	Decreased plasma levels
Penicillin, Methotrexate	Probenecid	Elevated plasma levels
Digoxin	Antibiotics	Increased Bioavailability

PROCEDURE

1. Prepare 0.02mM concentration of two drugs and a mixture of these drugs (each containing 0.02 mM).

2. Record the absorbance of drug solutions individually and for mixture at different wavelengths in a region (200 - 400 nm) with an increment of 10 nm.

3. Calculate the theoretical absorbance of mixture based on absorbance of individual drug solution using additive property.

4. Plot wavelength vs. absorbance values for drugs individually, mixture of drugs and theoretical values calculated by adding the absorbance values of two drugs on same graph paper and compare with practically observed absorbance values of the mixture.

Set up the following table for the obtained data:

Wave length	Drug A	Drug B	Mixture	Theoretical values (Drug A + Drug B)

REPORT

If the practically observed values are different from the expected theoretical values then there may be a possibility of drug-drug interaction.

EXPERIMENT 16

BIOAVAILABILITY AND
BIOEQUIVALENCE STUDIES

A Pharmaceutical Research Development group, have developed three different formulations (Tablets) of same drug. Then they have conducted the bioequivalence studies for all the three formulations and marketed formulation (Reference product/Innovator Product) using four way cross over design. Data obtained is given in the following table. Find out whether all formulations are bioequivalent to that of reference product or not by using Multiple ANOVA technique? (Refer Appendix 6)

Reference Product Code: A

Test Products Codes: B, C and D

Subjects	AUC Values (µg. hr/ml)			
	Period I	Period II	Period III	Period IV
1	51 (A)	33 (C)	53 (D)	32 (B)
2	33 (C)	53 (A)	35 (B)	54 (D)
3	52 (A)	34 (B)	35 (C)	55 (D)
4	36 (B)	55 (A)	56 (D)	37 (C)
5	35 (C)	37 (B)	57 (A)	58 (D)
6	37 (B)	35 (C)	54 (D)	58 (A)
7	52 (A)	53 (D)	36 (B)	35 (C)
8	54 (D)	56 (A)	36 (C)	33(B)
9	55 (D)	36 (B)	56 (A)	32 (C)
10	32 (B)	56 (D)	33 (C)	54 (A)
11	35 (C)	53 (A)	37 (B)	56 (D)
12	54 (A)	36 (C)	57 (D)	36 (B)
13	37 (B)	58 (D)	52 (A)	34 (C)
14	56 (D)	35 (B)	36 (C)	52 (A)
15	52 (D)	33 (C)	31 (B)	52 (A)
16	31 (C)	57(D)	54 (A)	33 (B)
17	34 (B)	57 (A)	58 (D)	32 (C)
18	55 (A)	36 (B)	35 (C)	52 (D)
19	51 (D)	37 (C)	57 (A)	37 (B)
20	39 (C)	57 (D)	32(B)	55 (A)
21	53 (D)	38 (B)	38 (C)	54 (A)
22	32 (B)	55 (D)	57 (A)	37 (C)
23	57 (A)	32 (C)	56 (D)	36 (B)

EXPERIMENT 17

DETERMINATION OF CREATININE CLEARANCE BY NOMOGRAM METHOD (HEIGHT)

AIM

Determination of creatinine clearance by using given nomogram (Height)

INTRODUCTION

Clearance is the theoretical concept for describing drug elimination from the body. It is defined as the hypothetical volume of the body fluid from which the drug is removed or cleared completely in a specific period of time. It is expressed in ml/min or liters/hr.

Clearance (CL) = Elimination rate/Plasma drug concentration

Creatinine is an endogenous amine and is a metabolic breakdown product of muscle creatinine phosphate. Creatinine clearance represents the rate at which creatinine is removed from blood by the kidneys. Creatinine production in an individual varies with age, weight, sex of the individual.

A direct method for determining creatinine clearance is determination of the amount of creatinine excreted in urine in 24 hrs and the mean of serum creatinine from blood samples taken just before and immediately after the urine collection period, following formula is used:

CL_{cr} = Rate of creatinine excretion/ Serum creatinine in mg

The normal creatinine clearance value is 120-130 ml/min. A value of 20-50 ml/min denote moderate renal failure and values below 10 ml/min indicate severe renal impairment.

The renal function, RF is calculated by,

RF = CL_{cr} of patient / CL_{cr} of a normal person

TRAUB and JOHNSON method uses a nomogram which requires the height and serum creatinine concentration of the patient. According to

39

the authors of this method, the development of this nomogram was based up on the observation of 81 children between the ages of 6 and 12 years.

Nomogram consists of 3 vertical lines, drawn parallel to each other and at the suitable distances from each other. These straight lines are as follows.

1. The vertical line on the left represents serum creatinine concentration. This straight line is subdivided into units expressing serum creatinine concentration in mg/100 ml. (or) mg/dL.

2. The vertical line on the right represents the height. This straight line is subdivided into units (cm). The height of the child in centimeters.

3. The vertical line in the middle of these two lines represents creatinine clearance. This straight line is subdivided into units and express creatinine clearance in ml/min/1.73 m^2.

PROBLEM

A child has a height of 80 cm with serum creatinine level of 1 mg/dL. Find out the creatinine clearance (CL$_{cr}$) using given nomogram?

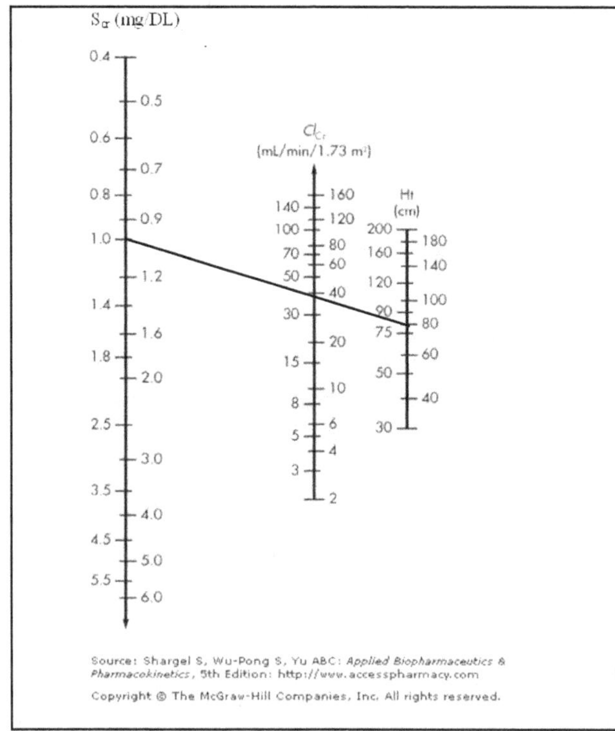

Construction of a Nomogram

Draw a straight line to connect the patient's serum creatinine value (mg/dL) to the patient's height. The point of intersection of this straight line and the vertical line in the middle of nomogram indicates creatinine clearance of the patient in ml/min/1.73 m^2.

REPORT

The creatinine clearance of child in above problem is 40 ml/min/1.73 m^2.

DETERMINATION OF CREATININE CLEARANCE BY NOMOGRAM METHOD (WEIGHT)

AIM

To determine the creatinine clearance by using nomograms (weight, age, gender, serum creatinine)

INTRODUCTION

Creatinine clearance represents the rate at which creatinine is removed from blood by the kidneys

$$CL_{cr} = \text{Rate of creatinine excretion} / \text{serum creatinine in mg.}$$

NOMOGRAM

- The Siersbask-Nielsen method used to determine the creatinine clearance by using a nomogram. The use of nomogram is relatively easier than using an equation.
- The nomogram consists of five vertical lines drawn parallel to and at suitable distances from each other. These lines are labeled as follows from left to right.
- Clearance (ml/min), weight (kg), R(no units, because this line represents the point of reference), Age (years) and serum creatinine (mg/100 ml)
- The vertical line labeled "age" is marked separately for males and females. The marking on the right side of this line are for females and markings on the left side are for males. The nomogram is used as follows.
    1. Draw a straight line to connect patient's weight (on the second line from left) to the patient's age (on the second line from right). This gives a point of intersection on the middle line 'R'

2. Draw a straight line to connect the patient's serum creatinine value on the first line on right to the point of intersection on line 'R' and extrapolate this straight line to the first line on left to read creatinine clearance.

Model Problem

Find out the creatinine clearance for an adult 45 years female weighing 65 kg having the serum creatinine levels as 3mg per 100 ml?

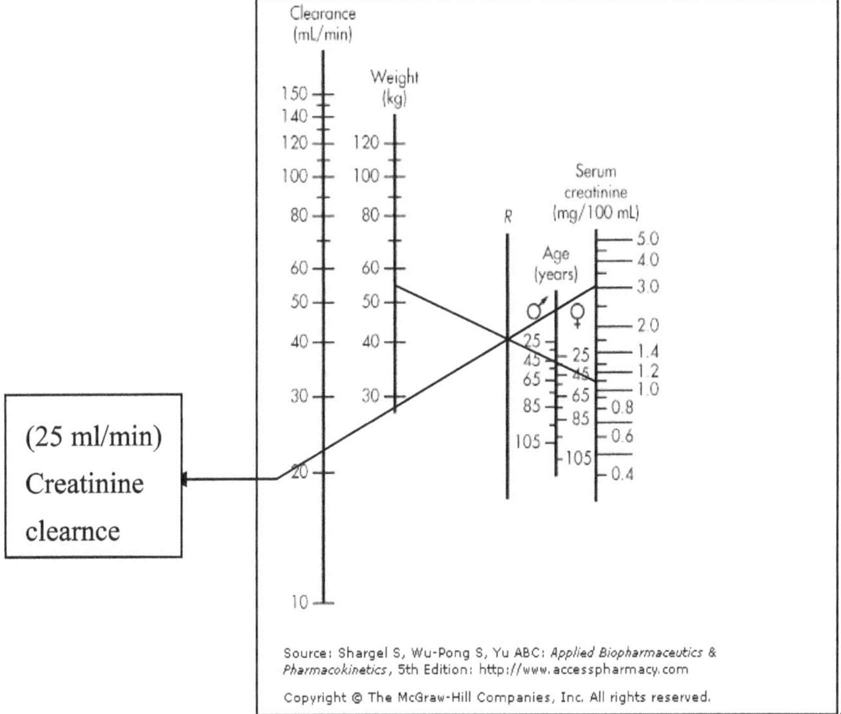

Normal method of estimation:

$$CL_{cr} = [140\text{-age (years)}] \times \text{Body weight (kg)} / [72 \times Cr_s \text{ (mg/dL)}]$$

$$= (140\text{-}45) \times 65 / (72 \times 3) = 6175/216 = 28.58\text{ml/min (males)}$$

Females $= 0.9 \times CL_{cr}$ of males $= 28.58 \times 0.9 = 25.72$ ml/min (approximately same as nomogram method)

REPORT

Creatinine clearance of women was calculated by nomogram and it was found to be 25.00 ml/min approx.

ONE COMPARTMENT OPEN MODEL-IV BOLUS

Model Problem

Enalapril is an ACE inhibitor used in the treatment of hypertension and CHF. The parent compound enalapril undergoes to a sole metabolite enalapril at which is more active than parent compound. A single 5 mg of IV dose of enalapril was administered to a 50 kg person and both plasma and urine samples were collected at various time intervals and analyzed for parent drug content.

The data obtained is given in following table

Time (Hrs)	Plasma Concentration (ng/mL)	Cumulative Amount of Drug Excreted in Urine (mg)
1	29	0.41
2	17	0.65
3	10	0.80
4	5.9	0.88
6	2	0.96

By using the above given data calculate all possible Pharmacokinetic Parameters by all three methods?

Assumption: The drug follows One Compartment Open Model

Note: (Refer Appendix 8 for detailed procedure)

I. Determination of Pharmacokinetic Parameters in Plasma:

Step 1: Plot the graph on semilogarthmic graph paper by taking concentration on Y axis and time on X axis which is shown below. A straight line is obtained. Extrapolate the straight line on to y axis. And calculate all the parameters by using the formulae given above.

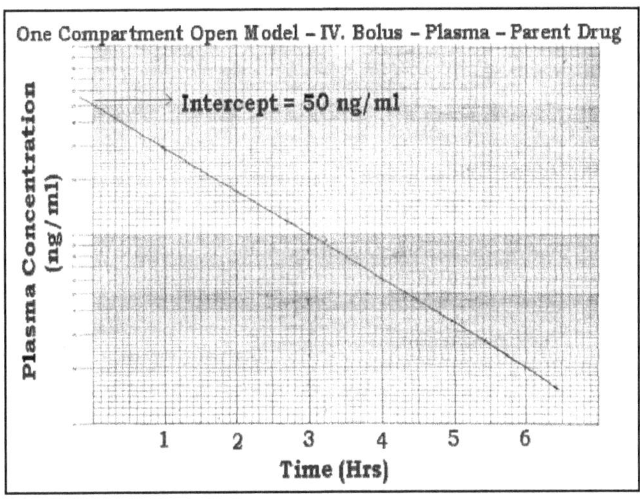

Step 2: **Estimation of pharmacokinetic parameters**

1. Intercept obtained is C_0=50 ng/mL

2. Slope of straight line = [log(5.9)–log(2)]/(4 – 6) = – 0.235

3. Apparent overall elimination rate constant (K) = –(– 0.235) × 2.303
    = 0.541/h

4. Elimination Half – Life $t_{1/2}$ (h) = 0.693/0.541 = 1.28 h

5. Apparent Volume of Distribution V_d (L) = 5 mg / 50 (ng/mL) =
    5000 × 1000ng/50 (ng/mL) = 100000 mL = 100 L

6. Area Under the Curve (AUC_0^{∞}) (µg.h/mL) = AUC_0^t + AUC_t^{∞}

    AUC_0^t (Trapezoidal Rule) (µg.h/mL) =

    $[(C_0 + C_1)/2] (t_1{-}t_0) + [(C_1{+} C_2)/2] (t_2{-}t_1) + {-}{-}{-}{-}+ [(C_{n-1}{+} C_n)/2] (t_n{-} t_{n-1})$

    AUC_t^{∞} (Integration Method) (µg.h/mL) = C_{last} / K

Time (h) (1)	Plasma Concentration (ng/mL) (2)	(Cn+Cn+1)/2 (3)	tn-tn-1 (4)	Area under each trepezoid (ng.h/mL) (5) = (3)*(4)
0	50	--	--	--
1	29	39.5	1	39.5
2	17	23	1	23
3	10	13.5	1	13.5
4	5.9	7.95	1	7.95
6	2	3.95	2	7.9
AUC_0^t				91.85

$$AUC_t^\infty = 2/0.541 = 3.696 \text{ ng.h/mL}$$

$$AUC_0^\infty = 91.85 + 3.696 = 95.54 \text{ ng.h/mL}$$

7. AUC_0^∞ (Integration Method) (μg.h/mL) = C_0 / K = 50/0.541 =

= 92.42 ng.h/mL

(AUC is Approxmately equal in both methods)

8. Area Under the Mean Curve $AUMC_0^\infty$ (μg.h^2/mL) = $AUMC_0^t$ + $AUMC_t^\infty$

$AUMC_0^t$ (Trapezoidal Rule) (μg.h^2/ml) =

$[(C_0t_0 + C_1t_1)/2]\ (t_1 - t_0) + [(C_1\ t_1 + C_2\ t_2)\ /2](t_2 - t_1) + \text{----} + [(C_{n-1}\ t_{n-1} + C_n\ t_n)/2](t_n - t_{n-1})$

$AUMC_t^\infty$ (μg.h^2/mL) = $[C_{last}\ t_{last}/K] + C_{last}/K^2$

Time (h) (1)	Plasma Concentration (ng/mL) (2)	$C_n t_n$ (3) = (1)*(2)	$(C_{n-1}\ t_{n-1} + C_n\ t_n)/2$ (4)	$t_n - t_{n-1}$ (5)	Area under each trepezoid (ng.h^2/mL) (6) = (4)*(5)
0	50	0	--	--	--
1	29	29	14.5	1	14.5
2	17	34	31.5	1	31.5
3	10	30	32	1	32
4	5.9	23.6	26.8	1	26.8
6	2	12	17.8	2	35.6
$AUMC_0^t$					140.4

$AUMC_t^\infty = [12/0.541] + [2/(0.541)^2] = 22.18 + 6.83 = 29.01 \text{ ng.h}^2/\text{mL}$

$AUMC_0^\infty$ (μg.h^2/mL) = $AUMC_0^t$ + $AUMC_t^\infty$ = 140.4 + 29.01 = 169.41 ng.h^2/mL

9. $AUMC_0^\infty$ (Integration Method) (μg.h^2/mL) = C_0 / K^2 = 50/(0.541)^2 = 170.83 ng.h^2/mL

(AUMC by both the methods are approximately equal)

10. Mean Residence Time (h) = $AUMC_0^\infty$/ AUC_0^∞ = 169.41/95.54 = = 1.77 h

Mean Residence Time (h) = 1/K = 1.84 h

(MRT by both methods approximately equal)

11. Total clearance CL_T (L/h) = Dose / AUC_0^∞

= 5 × 1000 × 1000 ng/95.54 ng.h/mL = 52334.1 mL/h = 52.33 L/h

Total clearance CL_T (L/h) = V_d . K = 100 × 0.541 = 54.1 L/h

(Total clearance by both the methods approximately equal)

2. Determination of Pharmacokinetic Parameters in urine by Excretion Rate method:

Step1: Computation of table

Time (hrs)	X_u^t (mg)	ΔX_u (mg)	Δt (h)	$\Delta X_u/\Delta t$ (mg/h)	Mid point of time t*(h)
1	0.41	0.41	1	0.41	0.5
2	0.65	0.24	1	0.24	1.5
3	0.80	0.15	1	0.15	2.5
4	0.88	0.08	1	0.08	3.5
6	0.96	0.08	2	0.04	5

Step 2: Plot the graph on semilogarthmic graph paper by taking $\Delta X_u/\Delta t$ on Y axis and mid point of time (t*) on X axis which is shown below. A straight line is obtained. Extrapolate the graph on to Y axis.

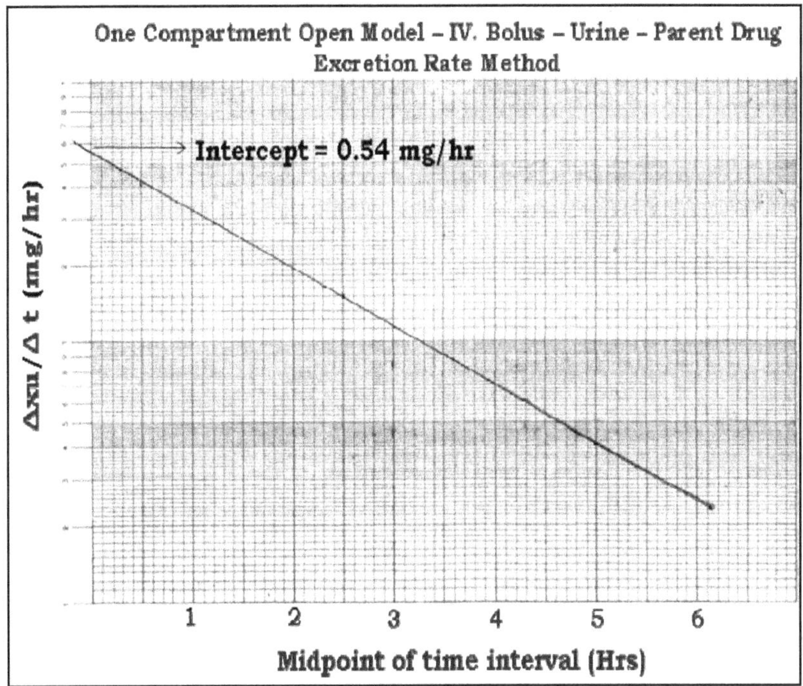

Step 3: Calculate the all possible pharmacokinetic parameters by using above mentioned formulae.

1. Intercept = KeX_0 (mg/h) = 0.54 mg/h

2. Slope $= [\log(0.41) - \log(0.24)]/(0.5-1.5) = (\times\, 0.387 + .619)/-1 =$
   -0.232

3. Overall Elimination Rate Constant $K(\,h^{-1}) = -(-0.232) \times 2.303 =$
   $0.534/h$

4. Elimination Half-Life $t_{1/2}$ (h) $= 0.693/K = 1.29$ h

5. Renal Excretion Rate Constant $(Ke)\,(\,h^{-1}) = $ Intercept $/X_0 = 0.54/5$
   $=0.108/hr$

6. Non Renal Excretion Rate Constant $(Ky)\,(h^{-1}) = 0.534 - 0.108 =$
   $0.426/h$

7. Renal Clearance CL_R (L/h) $= V_d\,.K_e = 100 \times 0.108 = 10.8$ L/h

8. Non Renal Clearance CL_{NR} (L/h) $= V_d\,.K_y = 100 \times 0.426$
   $= 42.6$ L/h

9. Total Clearance CL_T (L/h) $= CL_R + CL_{NR} = 10.8 + 42.6$
   $= 53.4$ L/h

10. Total Clearance CL_T (L/h) $= V_d\,K = 100 \times 0.534 = 53.4$ L/h

11. Fraction unchanged dose that ultimately excreted through renal pathway $f_e = 0.108/0.534 = 0.202$

12. Amount unchanged dose that ultimately excreted through renal pathway

$$X_u^{\infty} = 0.202 \times 5 = 1.02 \text{ mg}$$

3. Determination of Pharmacokinetic Parameters in urine by Sigma Minus method

Step 1: Computation of table

Time (hrs)	$X_u^{\,t}$ (mg)	$X_u^{\infty} - X_u^{\,t}$ (mg)
0	0	0.96
1	0.41	0.54
2	0.65	0.31
3	0.80	0.16
4	0.88	0.08
6	0.96 (X_u^{∞})	--

Step 2: Plot the graph on semilogarthmic graph paper by taking $X_u^{\infty} - X_u^{\,t}$ on Y axis and time on X axis which is shown below. A straight line is obtained.

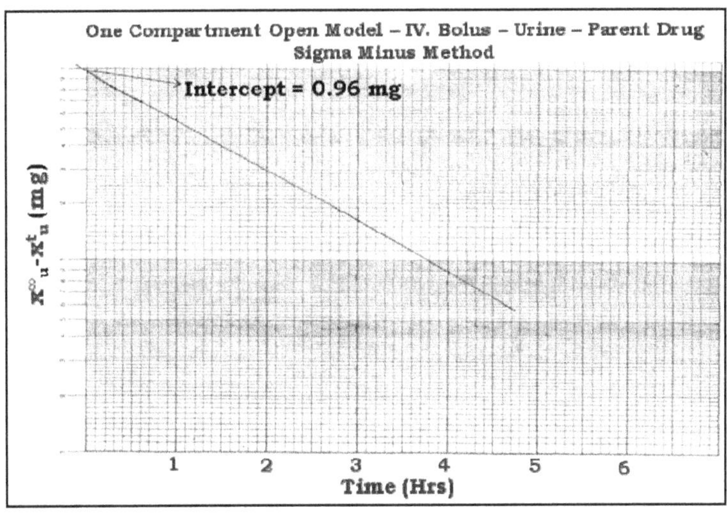

Step 3: Calculate the all possible pharmacokinetic parameters by using above mentioned formulae.

1. Intercept $= X_u^{\infty} = KeX_0 / K$ (mg) $= 0.96$ mg

2. Slope $= [\log(0.96) - \log(0.54)]/(0 - 1) = (-0.017 + 0.267) / -1 = -0.25$

3. Overall Elimination Rate Constant K $(h^{-1}) = (-0.25) \times 2.303 = 0.575$ h

4. Elimination Half-Life $t_{1/2}$ (h) $= 0.693 / 0.575 = 1.205$ h

5. Renal Excretion Rate Constant (Ke) $(h^{-1}) = 0.96 \times 0.575/5 = 0.11/h$

6. Non Renal Excretion Rate Constant (Ky) $(h^{-1}) = 0.575 - 0.11 = 0.465/h$

7. Renal Clearance CL_R (L/h) $= 100 \times 0.11 = 11$ L/h

8. Non Renal Clearance CL_{NR} (L/h) $= 100 \times 0.465 = 46.5$ L/h

9. Total Clearance CL_T (L/h) $= 11+46.5 = 57.5$ L/h

10. Total Clearance CL_T (L/h) $= 100 \times 0.575 = 57.5$ L/h

11. Fraction unchanged dose that ultimately excreted through renal pathway $f_e = 0.11/0.575 = 0.191$

12. Amount unchanged dose that ultimately excreted through renal pathway $X_u = 0.191 \times 5 = 0.956$ mg ≈ 0.96 mg

Practice Problems

1. A single IV dose 1000 mg of antibiotic was given to 50 kg women. Urine & blood samples were collected periodically & assayed for parent drug. From given data calculate all possible Pharmacokinetic parameters by 3 methods.

Time (hrs)	Plasma conc (ng/mL)	Urine vol (mL)	Conc of unchanged drug in urine(mg/mL)
0	?	250	0
0.25	4200	280	0.5714
0.50	3500	300	0.4666
1	2500	350	0.5714
2	1250	450	0.555
4	310	480	0.3917
6	80	360	0.1278

2. Metaprolol is used in the treatment of hypertension. The unchanged parent drug is excreted in urine. The following data is obtained upon administration of 200 mg IV bolus. Calculate all possible Pharmacokinetic parameters by 3 methods

Time (hrs)	Plasma conc (μg/mL)	Urine collection Interval (h)	X_u (mg)
0.5	0.364	0-1	1.82
1	0.331	1-2	1.5
2	0.274	2-3	1.28
4	0.187	3-5	0.94
6	0.128	5-7	0.64
8	0.088	7-13	0.52

3. A dose of 300 mg of new drug is injected IV to a healthy volunteer & the following blood data is obtained. Assume that the drug follows one compartment open model. Calculate all possible Pharmacokinetic parameters?

Time (h)	2	4	6	8	10	12	16
Plasma conc (μg/mL)	18.3	10.1	5.8	3.3	1.8	1	0.31

4. The following plasma data is obtained after an IV bolus dose of 200 mg 4th generation cephalosporin. Estimate all possible pharmacokinetic parameters?

Time (h)	1	6	12	24	48	72	96	144
Plasma conc (mg/L)	137	120	103	76	42	23	12	3.7

5. Plasma conc of cocaine after a single IV dose of 33 mg in a 75 kg male are given below Calculate all possible pharmacokinetic parameters?

Time (h)	0.16	0.5	1	1.5	2	2.5	3
Plasma conc (mg/L)	170	122	74	45	28	17	10

6. A 50 kg woman is given IV dose of an antibacterial drug at a dose level of 6 mg /kg Blood samples are taken at various time intervals. The conc. of the drug is determined in the plasma fraction of each blood sample & the following data were obtained:

Time (h)	0.25	0.5	1	3	6	12	18
Plasma conc. (mg/mL)	8.21	7.87	7.23	5.15	3.09	1.11	0.40

   1. What are the values of V_d, K and $t_{1/2}$ for this drug?

   2. This antibacterial agent is not effective at a plasma conc of less than 2 mg/ml. what is   the duration of activity for this drug?

   3. How long would it take for a 99.9% of this drug to be eliminated?

   4. If the dose of the antibiotic is doubled exactly, what be the increase in duration of activity?

7. A new antibiotic drug is given in a single IV bolus of 5 mg/kg to a healthy human volunteer (70 kg). The plasma level and time curve for this drug fits in to one compartment open model. The equation of the curve that best fits the:

$$C = 70 \ e^{-0.43t}$$

Determine the following (assume units of µg/ml for 'C' and hrs for 't':

   (a) What is the $t_{1/2}$?

   (b) What is the V_d?

   (c) What is the plasma level of the drug after 5 hrs?

(d)   How much drug is left in the body after 5 h?

(e)   Assuming the drug is no longer effective when levels decline to less than 2 mg/mL when would you administer the next dose?

8. An antibiotic is administered to a male adult suffering from UTI by an IV bolus (300 mg). The patient is instructed to empty his bladder prior to being medicated & to save his urine specimens for analysis. The urine samples are analyzed for drug content. The drug assays gave the following results:

Time(h)	0	4	8
Amt of drug in urine(mg)	0	100	26

Assuming 1st order elimination, calculate the elimination $t_{1/2}$ for the antibiotic in this patient.

EXPERIMENT 20

ONE COMPARTMENT OPEN MODEL-IV INFUSION

Model Problem

A drug has volume of distribution of 12 L and a K of 0.18 h^{-1}. A steady state concentration (C_{ss}) 12 mg/L is desired. (a). what is the infusion rate needed to maintain this concentration? (b)How long it takes to achieve 90% and 99% of the C_{ss}? (c)If the elimination rate constant, K, in a patient with a renal impairment is 0.1 h^{-1}, what is the infusion rate required maintaining the same C_{ss} in this patient?

Solution

(a) $C_{ss} = K_0 / KV_d$; $\qquad K_0 = C_{ss} KV_d = 12*0.18*12 = 25.92$ mg/h

(b) $Log (C_{ss} - C) = Log C_{ss} - Kt/2.303$

To achieve 90 % of C_{ss} : $C = 90C_{ss}/100$

$Log(10C_{ss}/100) = Log C_{ss} - Kt/2.303$

$Log(120/100) = Log(12) - 0.18t/2.303 \Rightarrow 0.079 = 1.079 - 0.18t/2.303$

$t = (1.079 - 0.079)*2.303/0.18 = 12.79$ h

To achieve 99 % of C_{ss} : $C = 99C_{ss}/100$

$Log(C_{ss}/100) = Log C_{ss} - Kt/2.303$

$Log(12/100) = Log(12) - 0.18t/2.303 \Rightarrow -0.92 = 1.079 - 0.18t/2.303$

$t = (1.079 + 0.92)*2.303/0.18 = 25.57$ h

(c) $K_0 = C_{ss} KV_d = 12*0.1*12 = 14.4$ mg/h

Practice Problems

1. A patient is given an antibiotic having $t_{1/2}$ of 4 hrs by constant IV infusion at a rate of 3 mg/h. At the end of 36 hrs, the plasma drug concentration is 2.2 mg/L. Calculate the total body clearance for this antibiotic. What is the volume of distribution, Vd, of the drug?

53

2. A patient is given an I.V infusion of an antibiotic at an infusion rate of 26 mg/h. Blood samples are taken at 10 and 28 hours and plasma drug concentrations are 10 and 11.9 mg/mL, respectively. The antibiotic has an elimination half life of 3 to 5 hrs in the general population. Estimate the elimination half life of the drug in this patient?

3. A drug whose $K = 0.02$ h^{-1} and $V_d = 20$ liters is infused to a patient at a rate of 3 mg/h for 8 h. What is the concentration of the drug in the body 2 h after the cessation of the infusion?

4. What is the concentration of a drug after 8 hours after administration of a loading dose of 100 mg and simultaneous infusion of 20 mg/h (the drug has a $t_{1/2}$ of 3 h and a volume of distribution 100 L)?

5. A doctor wants to maintain 2 mg/L of plasma drug level in a patient by administering a loading dose and simultaneously IV infusion to get Css of 2 mg/L. If the drug has an elimination rate constant, $K = 0.1$ h^{-1} and $V_d = 15$ L, What is the required loading dose and what is the required infusion rate?

6. An adult male patient (52 years, 70kg) is to be given an antibiotic by IV infusion. According to the literature, the antibiotic has an elimination half life of 2 hours, V_d of 0.9 L/kg, and is effective at a plasma drug concentration of 10 mg/L. The drug is supplied in 5 ml ampoules containing 200 mg/mL. Recommend a starting infusion rate in mg/h and mL/h?

7. An adult male asthmatic patient (78 kg, 48 years old) with a history of heavy smoking is given an IV infusion of aminophylline at a rate of 0.5 mg/kg per hour. A loading dose of 6 mg/kg was given by IV bolus injection just prior to the start of the infusion. At 2 hours after the start of the infusion, the plasma theophylline concentration is measured and found to contain 5.8 mg/mL. The apparent Vd for theophylline is 0.45 L/kg. Aminophylline is the ethylenediamine salt of theophylline and contains 80% theophylline base. Because the patient is responding poorly to the aminophylline therapy, the physician wants to increase the plasma theophylline concentration in the patient to 10 mg/mL. What dosage recommendation would you give to the physician? Would you recommend another loading dose?

8. A drug has elimination rate constant 0.02 h^{-1}, volume of distribution $= 20$ L, $K_o = 3$ mg/h. Infusion is continued for 8 hours. What is the concentration of drug in the body 2 hours after cessation of therapy? What is the amount of drug in the body 4 hours after cessation of therapy?

9. An antibiotic has a volume of distribution of 10 L and a K of 0.1 h^{-1}. A steady state plasma concentration of 10µg/mL is desired. Determine the infusion rate needed to maintain this concentration?

10. A patient was given an antibiotic ($t_{1/2}$ = 6 h) by constant IV infusion at a rate of 2 mg/h. At the end of 2 days, the serum drug concentration was 10 mg/L. Calculate the total body clearance for this antibiotic?

11. An antibiotic has an elimination half life of 3-6 h in the general population. A patient was given an IV infusion rate of 15 mg/h. Blood samples were taken at 8 and at 24 h and plasma drug concentrations were 5.5 and 6.5 mg/L, respectively. Estimate the elimination half life of the drug in this patient?

12. A physician wants to administer an anesthetic agent at a rate of 2 mg/h by IV infusion. The elimination rate constant is 0.1 h^{-1}, and the Vd is 10 L. What loading dose should be recommended if the doctor wants the drug level to reach 2µg/ml immediately?

13. What is the concentration of a drug 6 hours after administration of a loading dose of 10 mg and simultaneous infusion at 2 mg/h (the drug has a $t_{1/2}$ of 3 h and a V_d of 10 L)?

14. A patient was infused for 6 hours with a drug (k = 0.01 h^{-1}; Vd = 10 L) at a rate of 2 mg/h. What is the concentration of the drug in the body 2 hours after cessation of the infusion?

ONE COMPARTMENT OPEN MODEL-EXTRAVASCULAR

Model Problem

An antibiotic is administered orally to a healthy human volunteer (50 mg dose) and plasma samples are analyzed for parent drug. Calculate all possible pharmacokinetic parameters? Determine the absorption rate constant by wagner nelson method also?

Time (h)	0.5	1	1.5	2	3	4.5	6	8
C_p (µg/mL)	0.05	0.21	0.27	0.31	0.31	0.23	0.18	0.12

Solution

Step 1: Plot the graph on semilogarthmic paper by taking plasma concentration on Y axis and time on X axis as shown below. And compute the table

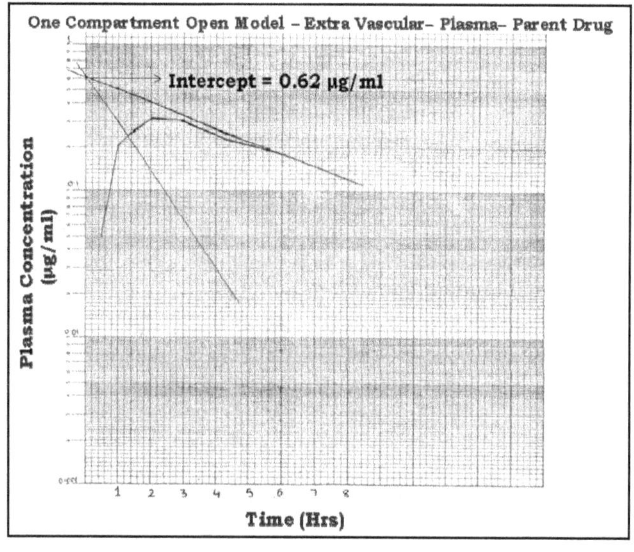

Time (h)	C_p (µg/mL)	Extrapolated conc. (C*)	Residual concentrations (C_r)
0.5	0.05	0.58	0.53
1	0.21	0.51	0.30
1.5	0.27	0.47	0.20
2	0.31	0.41	0.10
3	0.31	0.33	0.02
4.5	0.23	0.25	0.02
6	0.18	0.18	0
8	0.12	0.12	0

Step 2: Calculate all possible pharmacokinetic parameters by using above mentioned formulae.(Assume Ka>K)

1. Intercept $= (KaFX_0)/[V_d(Ka-K)]$ (µg/mL) $= 0.62$
2. Slope of extrapolated line $= [\log (0.18) - \log (0.12)]/ (6 - 8)$
   $= -0.088$
3. Slope of residual line $= [\log (0.27) - \log (0.02)]/ (1.5-4.5) = 0.376$
4. Overall elimination rate constant (K) $= -(-0.088) \times 2.303 = 0.202$/h
5. Elimination Half – Life of parent drug $t_{1/2}$ (h) $= 0.693/0.202 = 3.43$ h
6. Absorption rate constant $K_a(h^{-1}) = - (- 0.376) \times 2.303 = 0.865$/h
7. Absorption Half Life of drug $t_{1/2} = 0.693/ 0.865 = 0.801$ h
8. Area Under the Plasma – Time Curve AUC_0^{∞} (µg.h/mL)
   $= AUC_0^t + AUC_t^{\infty}$
   AUC_0^t (Trapezoidal Rule) (µg.h/mL) =

Time (Hs) (1)	C_p (µg/mL) (2)	$(C_n+C_{n+1})/2$ (3)	t_n-t_{n-1} (4)	Area under each trepezoid (µg.h/mL) (5) = (3)*(4)
0	0	--	--	--
0.5	0.05	0.025	0.5	0.0125
1	0.21	0.13	0.5	0.065
1.5	0.27	0.24	0.5	0.12
2	0.31	0.29	0.5	0.145
3	0.31	0.31	1	0.31
4.5	0.23	0.28	1.5	0.42
6	0.18	0.205	1.5	0.307
8	0.12	0.15	2	0.3
AUC_0^t (µg.h/mL) =				1.6795

AUC_t^{∞} (Integration Method) (µg.h/mL) $= C_{last} / K = 0.12/0.202 = 0.594$ µg.h/mL

AUC_0^{∞} (µg.h/mL) $= 1.6795 + 0.594 = 2.2735$ µg.h/mL

9. Area Under the Mean Curve $AUMC_0^\infty$ ($\mu g.h^2/mL$) = $AUMC_0^t$ + $AUMC_t^\infty$

    $AUMC_0^t$ (Trapezoidal Rule) ($\mu g.h^2/mL$)

    $AUMC_t^\infty$ ($\mu g.h^2/mL$) = $(C_{last} \, t_{last} / K) + (C_{last} / K^2)$

Time (h) (1)	C_p (μg/mL) (2)	$C_n t_n$ (3) = (1)*(2)	$(C_{n-1} t_{n-1} + C_n t_n)/2$ (4)	$t_n - t_{n-1}$ (5)	Area under each trepezoid (ng.h²/mL) (6) = (4)*(5)
0	0	0	--	--	--
0.5	0.05	0.025	0.0125	0.5	0.00625
1	0.21	0.21	0.1175	0.5	0.05875
1.5	0.27	0.405	0.3075	0.5	0.15375
2	0.31	0.62	0.512	0.5	0.256
3	0.31	0.93	0.775	1	0.775
4.5	0.23	1.035	0.982	1.5	1.473
6	0.18	1.08	1.057	1.5	1.5855
8	0.12	0.96	1.02	2	2.04
				$AUMC_0^t$	6.348

$AUMC_t^\infty$ = $(0.96 / 0.202) + 0.12 / (0.202)^2 = 7.692$ $\mu g.h^2/mL$

10. Mean Residence Time (h) = 7.692 /2.273 =3.384 h

    Mean Residence Time =1/K + 1/Ka = (1/0.202) + (1/0.865) = 6.1h

11. Volume of Distribution V_d (L) = 0.865 × 1 × 50/0.62 (0.865 − 0.202) = 105.23 L

12. Total clearance CL_T (L/h) = $V_d.K$ = 105.23 × 0.202 = 21.25L/h

    or FX0 / AUC = 50/2.273 =21.99 L/h

13. tmax = 2.303 log (0.865/0.202) /(0.865 − 0.202) = 2.193 h

14. Cmax = $50.e^{-0.202 \times 2.193}/105.23$ = 50 × 0.642/105.23 = 0.31μg/mL

Wagner Nelson-Method

Step 1: Compute the table

Time (h)	C_p (μg/mL)	$\int_0^t C \, dt$	$K \int_0^t C \, dt$	$C_p + K \int_0^t C \, dt$	$(A_\infty/V_d) - (A_t/V_d)$
0	0	--	--	--	--
0.5	0.05	0.0125	0.002	0.052	0.407
1	0.21	0.0775	0.015	0.225	0.234
1.5	0.27	0.1975	0.039	0.309	0.15
2	0.31	0.3425	0.069	0.379	0.08
3	0.31	0.6525	0.132	0.442	0.017
4.5	0.23	1.0725	0.216	0.446	0.013
6	0.18	1.3795	0.278	0.458	0.001
8	0.12	1.6795	0.339	0.459 (A_∞/V_d)	--

Step 2: Graph on semilogarthmic paper (shown below) by taking log percent unabsorbed $[(A_\infty/V_d) - (A_t/V_d)]$ on Y axis and time on X axis will givea a straight line with negative slope which is equivalent to absorption rate constant/2.303

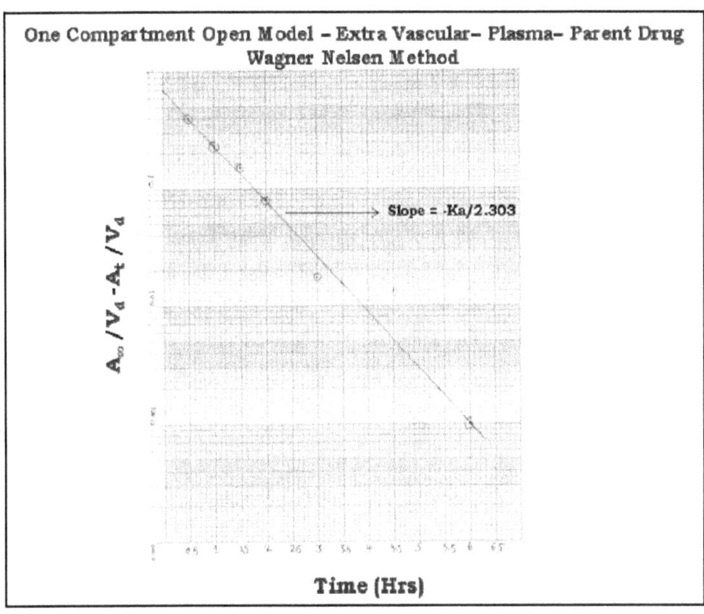

Step 3: Slope = [log(0.407)-log(0.15)]/0.5-1.5 = – 0.433

Step4: Absorption rate constant = – (–0.433) × 2.303 = 0.997/h

Practice Problems

1. Following plasma data is made available for various dosage forms of procainamide HCL (Dose 250mg).

Time (h)	Conc. of Procainamide base in µg/mL for		
	Tablet	**Capsule**	**IV Bolus**
0.33	0.68	0.26	-
0.5	0.82	0.67	-
0.66	1.17	0.93	-
1	1.23	1.12	1.45
1.33	1.31	1.19	1.35
2	1.39	1.12	1.18
3	0.93	0.96	0.95
4	0.74	0.74	0.77
6	0.51	0.51	0.51
8	0.32	0.30	0.33
12	0.11	0.09	0.14

1. Calculate all possible pharmacokinetic parameters?

2. Determine the absolute and relative bioavailability of different dosage forms?

3. How much drug will be excreted in urine (pH = 5.5) according to pH partition hypothesis?

   Note: Procainamide is a base (pKa = 9.1), as the HCL salt it is 87 % procainamide

2. A 59 kg male received 2 mg/kg of an antibiotic orally. The following plasma concentration versus time data is obtained. Assume the drug follows one compartment open model and is completely absorbed. Calculate all possible pharmacokinetic parameters. Determine absorption rate constant by Wagner nelson method also?

Time (h)	Plasma Concentration (µg/mL)
0.25	2.2
0.5	3.8
0.75	5
1	5.8
1.5	6.8
2	7.1
2.5	7.1
3	6.9
4	6.2
6	4.8
8	3.5
12	1.9
18	0.8
24	0.3

3. An antibiotic is administered orally to a healthy human volunteer (500 mg dose) and plasma samples are analyzed for parent drug. Calculate all possible pharmacokinetic parameters. Determine absorption rate constant by Wagner nelson method also?

Time (h)	C_p (µg/mL)
0.25	0.6
0.5	1.2
0.75	1.8
1	2.3
1.5	3.4
2	4.3

Table *Contd....*

Time (h)	C_p (µg/mL)
3	6.0
6	5.6
12	2.3
18	0.9
24	0.4

4. A drug is injected intramuscularly to a healthy human volunteer and the following plasma data is obtained. Determine absorption rate constant for the following data?

Time (h)	C_p (µg/mL)
0.5	2.4
1	3.8
1.5	4.2
2	4.6
4	8.1
6	5.8
10	5.1
16	4.1
24	3.0
32	2.3
48	1.3

5. pharmacokinetinetist gives griseofulvin orally, 0.5 g of a micronized drug formulation and, on another occasion intravenously, 100 mg to volunteers. The plasma concentration time data obtained in one subject are given below.

Time (h)	Plasma concentration of griseofulvin (mg/L)	
	IV Bolus	Oral Route
1	1.4	0.4
2	1.1	0.95
3	0.98	1.15
4	0.90	1.15
5	0.80	1.05
7	--	1.20
8	0.68	1.20
12	0.55	0.90
24	0.37	1.05
28	--	0.90
32	0.24	0.85
35	--	0.80
48	0.14	0.50

From appropriate plots and calculations, what can be calculated from these data with respect?

(a) Rate of absorption of griseofulvin with time on oral administration in this individual?

(b) Completeness of absorption?

6. A scientist measures phenytoin concentrations after the administration of sodium phenytoin intramuscularly (500mg) and intravenously (250 mg). The average data obtained in 12 subjects, each of whom received both treatments, are listed below.

Time (h)	Plasma concentration of Phenytoin (mg/L)	
	IM	IV
0	0	5.6
1	3.0	5.4
2	3.2	5.2
4	3.5	4.9
6	3.2	--
8	3.6	3.9
12	3.8	3.2
24	4.1	2.2
48	3.2	0.88
72	1.6	0.42

(a) Estimate the bioavailability of phenytoin from the IM site based on the areas of comparisons?

(b) From an appropriate plot of the data, comment on the process limiting the decline of the plasma phenytoin concentration following IM administration?

7. Plasma conc. following IV & oral administration of 500 mg of an antibiotic to a subject are given below:

Time (h)	Plasma conc of IV bolus(mg/L)	Plasma conc of oral route(mg/L)
0.33	14.7	-
0.5	12.6	2.4
0.67	11	-
1	-	3.8
1.5	9	4.2
2	8.2	4.6
4	7.9	8.1
6	6.6	5.8
10	6.2	5.1
16	4.6	4.1
24	3.2	3

1. From a semi logarithmic plot of the plasma conc., estimate the elimination $t_{1/2}$ of antibiotic in the subject
2. Calculate the total AUC following IV and oral administration???
3. From the IV data, estimate the CL and V_d of antibiotic??
4. Calculate the oral bioavailability of the drug ???

TWO COMPARTMENT OPEN MODEL-IV BOLUS

Model Problem

Ciprofloxacin 250 mg IV Bolus was administered to a patient and the following plasma data was obtained. Calculate all relevant pharmacokinetic parameters. Assume that the drug follows two compartment open model where elimination occurs from the central compartment.

Time (h)	Conc. (mcg/mL)
0.25	5.38
0.5	4.33
0.75	3.5
1	2.91
1.5	2.12
2	1.70
2.5	1.43
3	1.26
4	1.05
5	0.90
6	0.8
7	0.7

Calculate α, β, A, B, C_0, K_{10}, K_{12}, K_{21}, V_c, Vd_{ss}, V_t, V_β, V_{exp}, V_{area}, AUC, CL, t_{max} in tissue compartment and amount of drug in tissue compartment when t = 2 h?

Step 1: Plot the graph on semilogarthmic paper by taking plasma concentration on Y axis and time on X axis as shown below. And compute the table

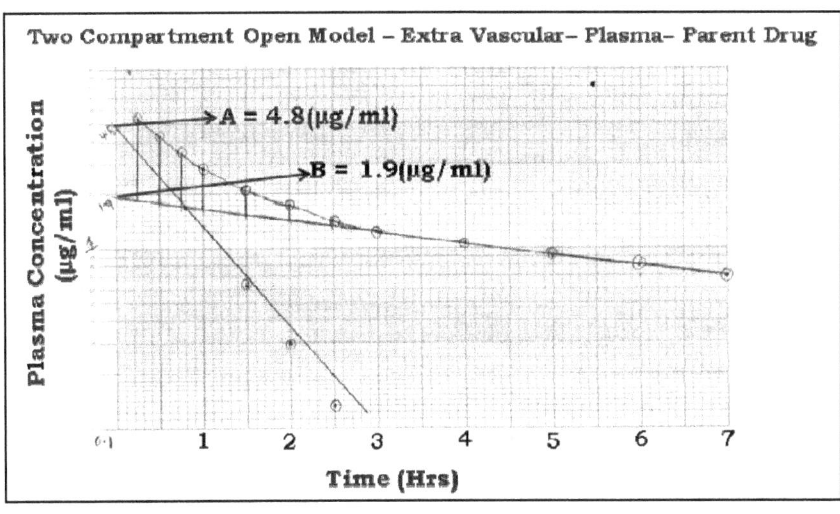

Time (h)	C_p (µg/mL)	Extrapolated conc. (C*)	Residual concentrations (C_r)
0.25	5.38	1.8	3.58
0.5	4.33	1.75	2.58
0.75	3.5	1.7	1.8
1	2.91	1.6	1.31
1.5	2.12	1.5	0.62
2	1.70	1.4	0.3
2.5	1.43	1.3	0.13
3	1.26	--	
4	1.05	--	
5	0.90	--	
6	0.8	--	
7	0.7	--	

1. Intercept of Extrapolated line = B = 1.9 µg/mL
2. Intercept of Residual line = A = 4.8 µg/mL
3. Slope of extrapolated line = [log (0.7) – log (0.8)]/ (7 –6) = – 0.058
4. Slope of residual line = [log (2.58) – log (3.58)]/ (0.5 – 0.25) = – 0.568
5. Rate constant of extrapolated line (β) = –(–0.058) × 2.303 (h^{-1}) = 0.133/h
6. Rate constant of residual line (α) = – (–0.568) × 2.303 (h^{-1}) = 1.308/h
7. Initial Plasma Concentration C_0 = A + B (µg/mL) = 1.9 + 4.8 = 6.7 µg/mL

8. K_{21} $(h^{-1}) = (\alpha B + \beta A) / (A + B) = 0.466/h$

9. K_{10} $(h^{-1}) = \alpha \beta / K_{21}$ (or) $[\alpha \beta(A+B)] / (\alpha B + \beta A) = 0.373/h$

10. K_{12} $(h^{-1}) = \alpha + \beta - K_{21} - K_{10}$ (or) $[AB (\alpha - \beta)^2] / [(A+B)(\alpha B + \beta A)]$
    $= 0.602/h$

11. Amount of the drug present in tissue compartment
    (X_t) $(mg) = (K_{12}X_0) (e^{-\beta t} - e^{-\alpha t})/ (\alpha - \beta) = 88.76$ mg

12. t_{max} in tissue compartment $= [2.303\log(\alpha/\beta)]/(\alpha - \beta) = 1.945$ h

13. Area Under the curve $= (A/\alpha) + (B/\beta) = 17.949$ µg.h/mL

14. Volume of distribution of Central Compartment $(V_c) = X_0/(A+B)$
    $= 37.31$ L

15. Volume of distribution at steady state $(Vd_{ss}) = [(K_{12} + K_{21})/K_{21}] V_c$
    $= 85.50$ L

16. Volume of distribution of tissue compartment $(V_t) = Vd_{ss} - V_c =$
    48.19 L

17. Volume of distribution by area $(Vd_{area}) = K_{10}.V_c / \beta$ (or) $X_0 / AUC.$
    $B = 104.63$ L

18. Volume of distribution by extrapolation $(Vd_{exp}) = X_0/ B = 131.57$ L

19. Clearance $= K_{10} \times V_c$ (or) $X_0 / AUC = 13.92$ L/h

20. $Vd_{exp} > Vd_{area} > Vd_{ss} > V_c$

Practice Problem

1. A dose of 100 mg of a drug is administered by rapid intravenous injection to a 70 kg healthy adult male. Blood samples are taken periodically after the administration of the drug and plasma fraction of each sample is assayed. The following data are obtained.

Time(H)	Plasma Concentration (mg/mL)
0.25	43
0.5	32
1	20
1.5	14
2	11
4	6.5
8	2.8
12	1.2
16	0.52

Assume that the drug follows a two compartment model and calculate all possible pharmacokinetic parameters?

EXPERIMENT 23

MULTIDOSE INJECTIONS

Model Problem

A subject receives 1000 mg every 6 hours by repetitive IV injections of an antibiotic with an elimination half life of 3 hours. Assume that the drug is distributed according to a one compartment open model and the volume of distribution is 20 L. Find the maximum, minimum and average plasma drug level. What are the loading and maintenance doses for this case?

Solution: Dosing interval $T = 6$ h; $V_d = 20$ L; $t_{1/2} = 3$ h; $K = 0.693/3 = 0.231/hr$

1. $R = e^{-kT}$ where T is the dosing interval $= e^{-(0.231)6} = 0.25$.
2. $C_{max} = C_1^0/ 1 - R = 50/1 - 0.25 = 50/0.75 = 66.66$ mg/L.
3. $C_{min} = R\, C_{max} = R\, (C_1^0/ 1 - R) = 16.67$ mg/L.
4. $C_{ave} = [AUC]_{t1}^{t2}/ T = X_0 / (V_d\, K\, T) = 36.1$ mg/L.
5. Loading Dose $X^* = C_{ave}\, V_d/ e^{-kT} = 2887.15$ mg.
6. Maintenance dose $= X^* (1 - R) = 2165.15$ mg.

67

MULTIDOSE EXTRAVASCULAR

Practice Problem

A male patient is given orally 250 mg of tetracycline HCl every 8 hours. The antibiotic absorption rate constant is 0.9 h^{-1} and the biological half life is 10 h. If the fraction of the dose absorbed is 0.75 and the volume of distribution is 121.5 L, calculate C_{max}, C_{min}, and C_{ave} at steady state. Find out the loading dose and maintenance dose for this case?

$t_{1/2} = 10$ h; $K = 0.693/10 = 0.0693/h$;

$T = 8h$; $V_d = 121.5$ L; $F = 0.75$; $Ka = 0.9/h$

$t_{max} = [2.303 \log(ka/k)]/(Ka - k) = 3.087$ h

$$C_{max} = \frac{KaFX_0}{V_d(Ka - K)}\left[\frac{e^{-Kt_{max}}}{1 - e^{-kT}} - \frac{e^{-Ka t_{max}}}{1 - e^{-kaT}}\right]$$

1. $C_{max} = 3.0675$ mg/L

2.

$$C_{min} = \frac{KaFX_0}{Vd(Ka - K)}\left[\frac{1}{1 - e^{-kT}} - \frac{1}{1 - e^{-kaT}}\right]$$

$C_{min} = 2.24$ mg/L.

3. $C_{ave} = FX_0 / (V_d K T) = 2.78$ mg/ L.

4. Loading Dose $X^* = (C_{ave} V_d / e^{-kT}) / F = 784$ mg.

5. Maintenance Dose $= X^* (1 - R) = 333.65$ mg.

APPENDIX 1

DEFINITIONS

BIOPHARMACEUTICS

Biopharmaceutics is defined as the study of factors influencing the rate and amount of drug that reaches the systemic circulation and the use of this information to optimize the therapeutic efficacy of the drug products.

DRUG ABSORPTION

Absorption is defined as the process of movement of unchanged drug from the site of administration to systemic circulation.

DRUG DISTRIBUTION

The reversible transfer of drug between one compartment and the other (generally blood and the extra vascular tissues) is referred to as drug distribution.

METABOLISM

Metabolism is defined as the conversion of drug from one chemical form to another chemical form. It is also called as biotransformation. Metabolism usually inactivates the drug.

EXCRETION

Excretion is defined as the irreversible removal of the drug from the body

ELIMINATION

Elimination is combination of metabolism and excretion.

DISPOSITION

Disposition is the combination of distribution, metabolism and excretion.

DISSOLUTION RATE

Dissolution rate is defined as the amount of solid substance that goes into solution per unit time under standard conditions of temperature, pH, solvent composition and constant solid surface area.

BIOAVAILABILITY

Bioavailability is defined as the rate and extent (amount) of drug that reaches systemic circulation or it is the rate and extent of drug absorption. It is of two types.

ABSOLUTE BIOAVAILABILITY

When the systemic availability of a drug administered orally (Extravascularly) is determined in comparison to its intravenous administration is called as absolute bioavailability.

Plasma:$\qquad$$F_{absolute} = [AUC_{EV} * Dose_{IV}] / [AUC_{IV} * Dose_{EV}]$

Urine:$\qquad$$[Xu^{\infty}_{EV} * Dose_{IV}] / [Xu^{\infty}_{IV} * Dose_{EV}]$

$\qquad\qquad\qquad$(EV-Extravascular; IV-Intravascular)

RELATIVE BIOAVAILABILITY

When the systemic availability of a drug after oral administration is compared with that of an oral standard of the same drug (such as an aqueous or non-aqueous solution or a suspension), it is referred to as Relative bioavailability.

Plasma:$\qquad$$F_{relative} = [AUC_T * Dose_R] / [AUC_S * Dose_T]$

Urine:$\qquad$$[Xu^{\infty}_T * Dose_R / [Xu^{\infty}_R * Dose_T]$

$\qquad\qquad\qquad$(T-Test; R-Reference)

CHEMICAL EQUIVALENCE

Two or more drug products are said to be chemical equivalent if they have the same labeled chemical substance as an active ingredient in the same amount.

PHARMACEUTICAL EQUIVALENCE

Two or more drug products are said to be pharmaceutical equivalent if they have same active ingredient, same strength, dosage form for same route of administration, but may differ in particle size of drug, excipients, method of manufacture. So all pharmaceutical equivalent products are need not be bioequivalent.

THERAPEUTIC EQUIVALENCE

Two or more drug products are said to be therapeutic equivalent if they have the same therapeutically active ingredient which elicits the same pharmacological effect to control the disease to the same extent.

BIOEQUIVALENCE

It is a relative term which denotes that the drug substance in two or more identical dosage forms, reaches the systemic circulation at the same relative rate and to the same relative extent i.e., their plasma concentration-time profiles will be identical without significant statistical differences.

PHARMACOKINETICS

Pharmacokinetics is defined as the kinetics of drug absorption, distribution, metabolism and excretion (KADME) and their relationship with the pharmacologic, therapeutic or toxicological response in man and animals.

CLINICAL PHARMACOKINETICS

The applications of pharmacokinetic principles in the safe and effective management of individual patient are called Clinical pharmacokinetics.

CHRONOKINETICS

A time dependent pharmacokinetics of drug is known as Chronokinetics or chronopharmacokinetics.

THERAPEUTIC DRUG MONITORING (TDM)

Management of drug therapy in individual patient often requires evaluation of response of the patient to the recommended dosage regimen. It is a branch of clinical chemistry and clinical pharmacology that specializes in the measurement of medication concentrations in blood. Its main focus is on drugs with a narrow therapeutic range, i.e., drugs that can easily be under- or overdosed. TDM aimed at improving patient care by individually adjusting the dose of drugs for which clinical experience or clinical trials have shown it improved outcome in the general or special populations.

LEVEL OF SIGNIFICANCE (LS)

It is an arbitrarily selected point in the probability scale, below which the probability is considered low, and equal to or above which the probability is considered high. Conventionally 0.05 (95% confidence interval) or 0.01 (99% confidence interval) of level of significance is used in biostatistics

DEGREES OF FREEDOM (DF)

The DF of a distribution is defined as the number of variates that can be entered in that distribution before the values of the remainder of the variates are fixed by the necessity to produce a certain total. Usually the degrees of freedom of any distribution is assumed as n-1 (n is total number of variables).

POLYMORPHISM

If any substance exists in more than one crystalline form is said to be polymorphism

COMPARTMENT

Compartment is defined as group of tissues which behaves similarly with respect to drug movement

APPENDIX 2

DISINTEGRATION

INTRODUCTION

Disintegration time (DT) is of particular importance in case of solid dosage forms like tablets and capsules. *In vitro* disintegration test is by no means a guarantee of drug's bioavailability because if the disintegrated drug particles do not dissolve, absorption is not possible. However, if a solid dosage form does not conform to the DT, it portends bioavailability problems because the subsequent process of dissolution will be much slower and absorption may be insufficient. Rapid disintegration is thus important in the therapeutic success of a solid dosage form. The state in which any residue of unit (tablet or capsule), except fragments of insoluble coating or capsule shell remain on the screen of test apparatus in a soft mass having no palpably firm core is considered as complete disintegration. Enteric coated tablets are meant to disintegrate in intestinal pH and should not show any signs of disintegration in acidic environment. Disintegration test determines whether the tablets or capsules disintegrate within a prescribed time when placed in a medium under the standard experimental conditions. If discs have been used with capsules, any residue remaining on the lower surfaces of the discs consists only of fragments of shells, not the firm core of unit. However, this test is not applicable to sustained release or controlled release tablets.

APPARATUS FOR DISTINTEGRATION OF TABLETS AND CAPSULES

1. Disintegration testing apparatus consists of a rigid basket- rack assembly supporting six cylindrical glass tubes, 77.5 ± 2.5 mm long, 21.5 mm in internal diameter and with a wall thickness of about 2 mm (see fig. 1)

2. The tubes are held vertically by two superimposed transparent plastic plates, 90 mm in diameter and 6 mm thick, perforated by six holes having the same diameter as the tubes.

73

3. The holes are equidistant from the centre of the plate and are equally spaced from one another.

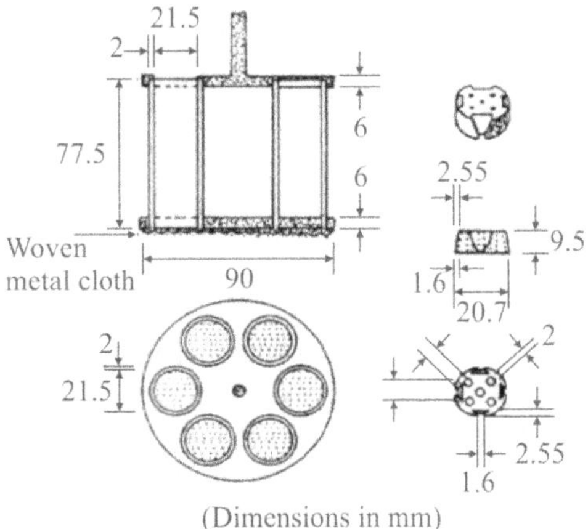

Fig 1 Disintegration testing apparatus.

4. Attached to the under side of the lower plate is a piece of woven gauze made from stainless steel wire 635 μm in diameter and having nominal mesh apertures of 2.00 mm (10mesh).

5. The plates are held rigidly in position and attached to a mechanical device capable of oscillating up and down smoothly at a constant frequency of **28 to 32 cycles per minute** through a distance of 50-60 mm. During upside movement, the wire mesh is suspended 25 mm in medium, similarly during downward movement the wire mesh is above 25 mm from bottom of beaker

6. A cylindrical disc for each tube, each 20.7 ± 0.15 mm in diameter and 9.5 ± 0.15 mm thick, made of transparent plastic with a relative density of 1.18 to 1.20, and pierced with five holes, each 2 mm in diameter, one in the centre and other four spaced equally on a circle of radius 6 mm from the centre of the disc.

7. The assembly is suspended in one liter beaker containing 900 ml of disintegrating medium. Disintegrating medium used may be water or 0.1 N HCL for all dosage forms except enteric coating dosage forms, where 0.1 N HCL or simulated gastric fluid used for first two hours and followed by 6.8 pH mixed phosphate buffer or simulated intestinal fluid is used for next one hour.

8. A thermostatic arrangement is present within the apparatus for heating the medium and temperature is maintained at **37°C ± 2°C.**

LIMITS OFFICIAL IN PHARMACOPOEIA

Uncoated tablets (IP): Not more than 15 min (In water). If 1 or 2 tablets fail to disintegrate completely repeat the test on 12 additional tablets. Not less than 16 of the total of 18 units tested disintegrate completely within specified time.

Film coated (IP): 30 min (In water). If 1 or 2 tablets fail to disintegrate completely repeat the test on 12 additional tablets. Not less than 16 of the total of 18 units tested disintegrate completely within specified time.

Sugar coated (IP): 60 min (In water). If 1 or 2 tablets fail to disintegrate completely repeat the test on 12 additional tablets. Not less than 16 of the total of 18 units tested disintegrate completely within specified time.

Enteric coated:

IP

Stage 1: Two hrs in gastric fluid (0.1 N HCl) - No evidence of disintegration, cracking or softening.

Stage 2: one hr in intestinal fluid (6.8 pH mixed phosphate buffer) – disintegrate completely.

If 1 or 2 tablets fail to disintegrate completely repeat the test on 12 additional tablets. Not less than 16 of the total of 18 units tested disintegrate completely within specified time.

USP

Stage 1: Simulated gastric fluid for 1 hour - No evidence of disintegration, cracking or softening.

Stage 2: simulated intestinal fluid for the time specified in the monograph - disintegrate completely. If 1 or 2 tablets fail to disintegrate completely repeat the test on 12 additional tablets. Not less than 16 of the total of 18 units tested disintegrate completely within specified time.

Dispersible Tablets (IP): NMT 3 min (In water).

Orodispersible Tablets **(Eur. Pharm.):** NMT 3 min.

Effervescent Tablets (IP): NMT 3 min (In water).

Hard Gelatin Capsules (IP): 30 min (In water).

Soft Gelatin Capsules (IP): 60 min (In water).

APPENDIX 3

DISSOLUTION

DEFINITION

Dissolution is defined as mass transfer from the solid surface to the liquid phase. Pharmaceutical solid dosage forms and dispersed systems form on administration undergo dissolution in biological media, followed by absorption of the drug entity into the systemic circulation.

DISSOLUTION RATE

Dissolution rate is defined as the amount of solid substance that goes into the solution per unit time under standard conditions of temperature, pH, solvent composition and constant solid surface area.

MECHANISM OF DISSOLUTION

Dissolution process in a solid dosage form is presented by wagner's model, and carstensen's model.

Wagner's Model

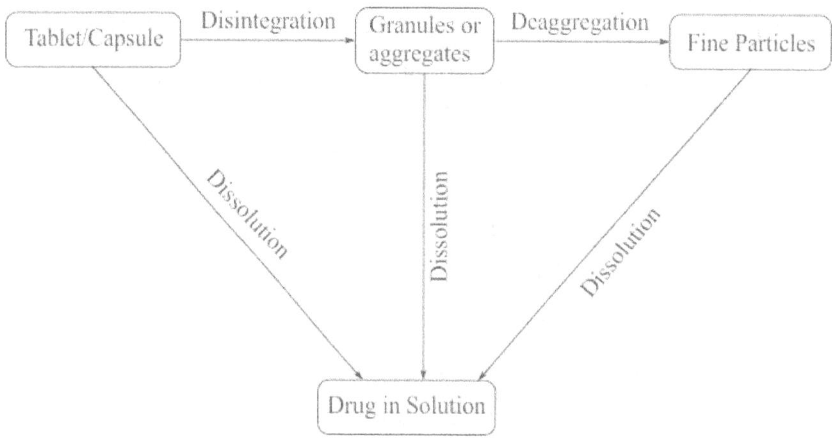

Fig. 1 Wagner's Dissolution

Carstensen's model

By the modification of Wagner's model to incorporate some other factors that proceed the dissolution process at solid dosage forms, Carstensen proposed a scheme incorporating the following sequence:

- Initial mechanical lag
- Wetting at the dosage forms
- Penetration of dissolution medium into the dosage form
- Disintegration
- Deaggregation
- Dissolution.

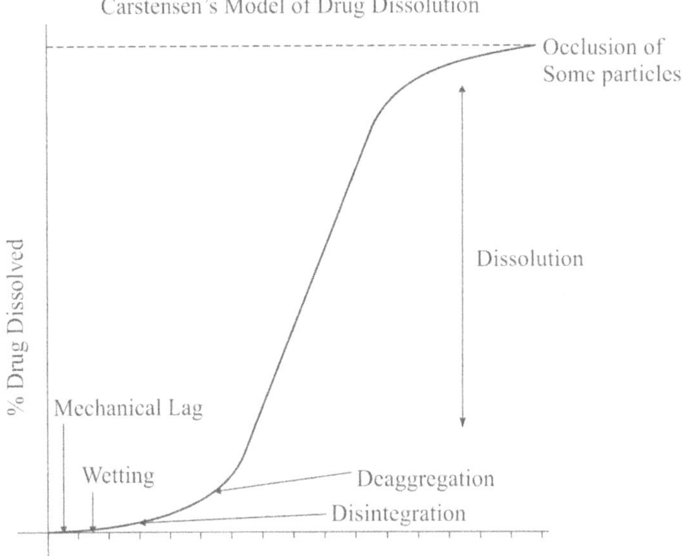

Fig. 2 Carstensen's Method of drug dissolution

THEORY

Dissolution is a dynamic process. Several theories were proposed to explain drug dissolution process. Some of the important ones are (Fig. 3):

1. Diffusion layer model/Film theory

2. Danckwert's model/Penetration or Surface renewal theory, and

3. Interfacial barrier model/Double barrier or Limited solvation theory.

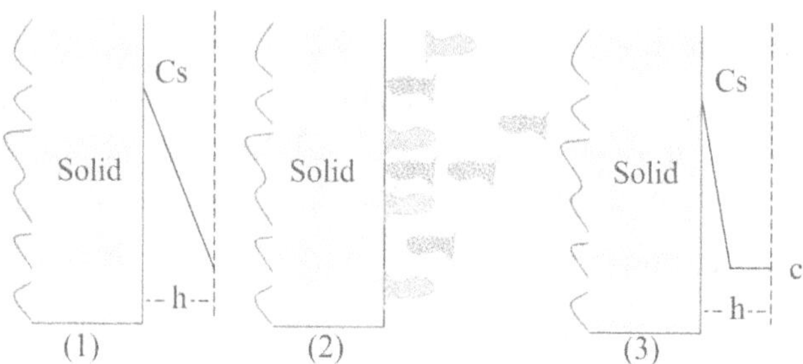

Fig. 3 Different theories of drug dissolution

The rate of dissolution when the process is diffusion controlled and involves no chemical reaction was given by modified Noyes-Whitney's (Brunner's) equation

$$\frac{dc}{dt} = \frac{DAK_{w/o}(c_s - c_b)}{Vh}$$

Where

D	=	diffusion coefficient of the drug
A	=	surface area of the dissolving solid
$K_{w/o}$	=	Water/Oil partition coefficient of the drug
V	=	volume of dissolution medium
h	=	thickness of the stagnant layer
(Cs-Cb)	=	concentration gradient for diffusion of drug

The above equation represents first-order dissolution rate process, the driving force for which is the concentration gradient (Cs-Cb). Under such a situation, dissolution is said to be under non-sink conditions. This is true in case of *in vitro* dissolution in a limited dissolution medium. Dissolution in such a situation slows down after sometime due to build-up in the concentration of drug in the bulk of the solution. The *in vivo* dissolution is always rapid than *in vitro* dissolution because the moment the drug dissolves it is absorbed into the systemic circulation. As a result $C_b = 0$, and dissolution is at its maximum. Thus, under *in vivo* conditions, there is no concentration build-up in the bulk of the solution and hence no retarding effect on the dissolution rate of the drug i.e. Cs >> Cb and sink conditions are maintained. To obtain good *in vitro-in vivo* dissolution rate correlation, the *in vitro* dissolution must always be carried under sink conditions. This can be achieved by:

1. Bathing the dissolving solid in fresh solvent from time to time

2. Increasing the volume of dissolution fluid

3. Removing the dissolved drug by partitioning it from the aqueous phase of the dissolution fluid into an organic phase placed either above or below the dissolution fluid. Ex. hexane or chloroform.

4. Adding a water miscible solvent such as alcohol to the dissolution fluid, or

5. By adding selected adsorbents to remove the dissolved drug

Note: *the in vitro sink conditions are so maintained that Cb is always less than 10% of Cs.*

OFFICIAL DISSOLUTION APPARATUS:

USP states 7 apparatus for dissolution testing of different dosage forms.

APPARATUS	NAME OF APPARATUS	DRUG PRODUCT
TYPE I	Rotating basket method	Tablets
TYPE II	Rotating paddle method	Tablets, capsules & modified drug products
TYPE III	Reciprocating cylinder	Extended-release drug products
TYPE IV	Flow through cell	Low water soluble drugs
TYPE V	Paddle over disk	Transdermal drug products.
TYPE VI	Cylinder	Transdermal drug products
TYPE VII	Reciprocating holder	Extended-release drug products/Transdermal drug products

NON - OFFICIAL DISSOLUTION APPARATUS:

1. Beaker - Stirrer Method
2. Flask – Stirrer Method
3. Rotating Bottle Method
4. Peristalsis Method
5. Static or Rotating Disk Method

DISSOLUTION TEST FOR TABLETS AND CAPSULES

1. Use Apparatus 2 unless otherwise directed.

2. All parts of the apparatus that may come into contact with the preparation being examined or with the dissolution medium are chemically inert and do not adsorb, react or interfere with the preparation being examined.

3.   All metal parts of the apparatus that may come into contact with the preparation or the dissolution medium must be made from stainless steel, type 316 or equivalent or coated with a suitable material to ensure that such parts do not react or interfere with the preparation being examined or the dissolution medium.

4.   No part of the assembly, including the environment in which the assembly is placed, contributes significant motion, agitation or vibration beyond that due to the smoothly rotating element

5.   An apparatus that permits observation of the preparation being examined and the stirrer during the test is preferable.

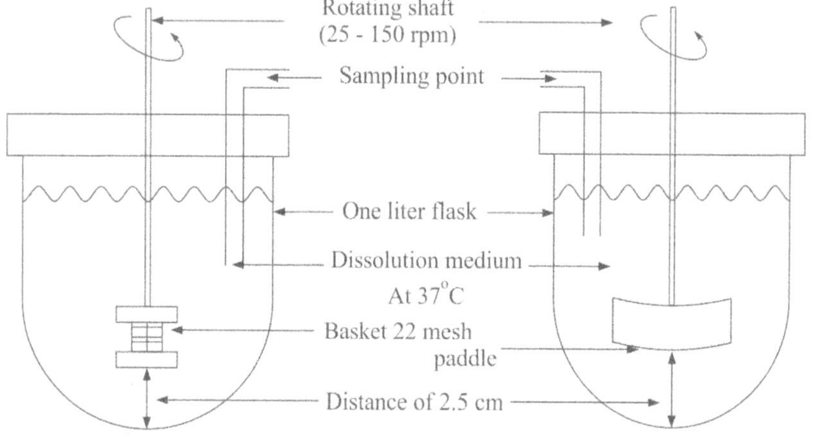

Fig. 4 Dissolution testing apparatus USP Type I and II

6.   Apparatus I:

(a) A cylindrical vessel, A, made of borosilicate glass or any other suitable transparent material, with a hemispherical bottom and with a nominal capacity of 1000 ml. The vessel has a flanged upper rim and is fitted with a lid that has a number of openings, one of which is central (see Fig. 4).

(b) A motor with a speed regulator capable of maintaining the speed of rotation of the basket within 4% of that specified in the individual monograph. The motor is fitted with a stirring element which consists of a drive shaft and blade forming a basket, D (see Fig. 4). The metallic shaft rotates smoothly and without significant wobble.

(c) The basket consists of two components. The top part, with a vent, is attached to the shaft C. it is fitted with three spring clips, or other suitable means, that allow removal of the lower part for introduction of the product/dosage form being examined and that firmly hold the lower part of the basket concentric with the axis of the vessel during rotation.

(d) The lower detachable part of the basket is made of welded-steam cloth, with a wire thickness of 0.254 mm diameter and with 0.381mm square openings, formed into a cylinder with narrow rim of sheet metal around the top and the bottom.

(e) The basket may be plated with a 2.5 mm layer of gold for use with acidic media. The distance between the inside bottom of the vessel and the basket is maintained at 23 to 27mm during the test

7. **Apparatus II:** An assembly consists of the following

(a) A cylindrical vessel, A, made of borosilicate glass or any other suitable transparent material, with a hemispherical bottom and with a nominal capacity of 1000 ml (see Fig. 4). The vessel has a flanged upper rim and is fitted with a lid that has a number of openings, one of which is central.

(b) A motor with a speed regulator capable of maintaining the speed of rotation of the paddle within 4% of that specified in the individual monograph. The motor is fitted with a stirring element which consists of a drive shaft and blade forming a paddle, B (see Fig. 4).

(c) The blade passes through the diameter of the shaft so that the bottom of the blade is flush with the bottom of the shaft. The shaft is positioned so that its axis is within 2 mm of the axis of the vessels and the lower edge of the blade is 23 to 27 mm from the inside bottom of the vessel. The apparatus operates in such a way that the paddle rotates smoothly and without significant wobble.

(d) Water -bath set to maintain the dissolution medium at 36.5° C to 37.5°C. The bath liquid is kept in constant and smooth motion during the test. The vessel is securely clamped in the water-bath in such a way that the displacement vibration from other equipment, including the water circulation device, is minimized.

8. **Dissolution Medium:** Use the dissolution medium specified in the individual monograph. If the medium is a buffered solution, adjust the solution so that its pH is within 0.05 units of the pH specified in the monograph. The dissolution medium should be deaerated prior to testing.

9. **Time:** Where a single time specification is given in the monograph, the test may be concluded in a shorter period if the requirement for the minimum amount dissolved is met. If two or more times are specified, specimen are to be withdrawn only at the stated times, within a tolerance of $\pm\ 2\%$.

10. **Method:** Introduce the stated volume of the dissolution medium, free from dissolved air, into the vessel of the apparatus. Warm the dissolution medium to between 36.5° and 37.5°C. Unless otherwise stated use one tablet or capsule.

11. When Apparatus 2 is used, allow the tablet or capsule to sink to the bottom of the vessel prior to the rotation of the paddle. A suitable device such as a wire of glass helix may be used to keep horizontal at the bottom of the vessel tablets or capsules that would otherwise float. Care should be taken to ensure that air bubbles are excluded from the surface of the tablet or capsule.

12. When Apparatus 1 is used, place the tablet or capsule in a dry basket at the beginning of each test. Lower the basket into position before rotation. Operate the apparatus immediately at the speed of rotation specified in the individual monograph.

13. Within the time interval specified, or at each of the times stated, withdraw a specimen from a zone midway between the surface of the dissolution medium and the top of the rotating blade or basket, not less than 10 mm from the wall of the vessel.

14. Except in the case of single sampling, add a volume of dissolution medium equal to the volume of the samples withdrawn.

15. Perform the analysis as directed in the individual monograph. Repeat the whole operation five times.

16. Where two or more tablets or capsules are directed to be placed together in the apparatus, carry out six replicate tests.

17. For each of the tablet or capsule tested, calculate the amount of dissolved active ingredient in solution as a percentage of the stated amount where two or more tablets or capsules are placed together, determine for each test the amount of active ingredient in solution

per tablet or capsules and calculate as a percentage of the stated amount.

18. If the results do not conform to the requirements at stage S1 given in the accompanying acceptance table (Table 1), continue testing with additional tablets or capsules through stages S2 and S3 unless the result conform at stage S2.

19. Where capsule shells interfere with the analysis, remove the contents of not less than 6 capsules as completely as possible, and dissolve the empty capsule shells in the specified volume of the dissolution medium. Perform the analysis as directed in the individual monograph. Make any necessary correction. Correction factors should not be greater than 25% of the stated amount

Table 1 Acceptance Table

STAGE	TABLETS TESTED	ACCEPTANCE CRITERIA
S1	6	Each unit is not less than D* + 5%
S2	6	Average of 12 units (S1 +S2) is equal to or greater than D, and no unit is less than D - 15%.
S3	12	Average of 24 units (S1+S2+S3)is equal to or greater than D, not, More than 2 units are less than D - 15% and no unit is less than D - 25%

*D is the amount of dissolved active ingredient specified in the individual monograph, expressed as a percentage of the stated amount.

USP APPARATUS III (RECIPROCATING CYLINDER):-

PRINCIPLE AND DESIGN

1. The development of USP Apparatus 3 was based on the recognition of the need to establish IVIVC, since the dissolution results obtained with USP Apparatuses I and II may be significantly affected by the mechanical factors such as shaft wobble, location, centering, deformation of the baskets and paddles, presence of the bubbles in the dissolution medium, etc.

2. The design of the USP Apparatus III (which is often referred to as the ''Bio-Dis.''), based on the disintegration tester, additionally incorporates the hydrodynamic features from the rotating bottle method and provides capability agitation and media composition changes during a run as well as full automation of the procedure.

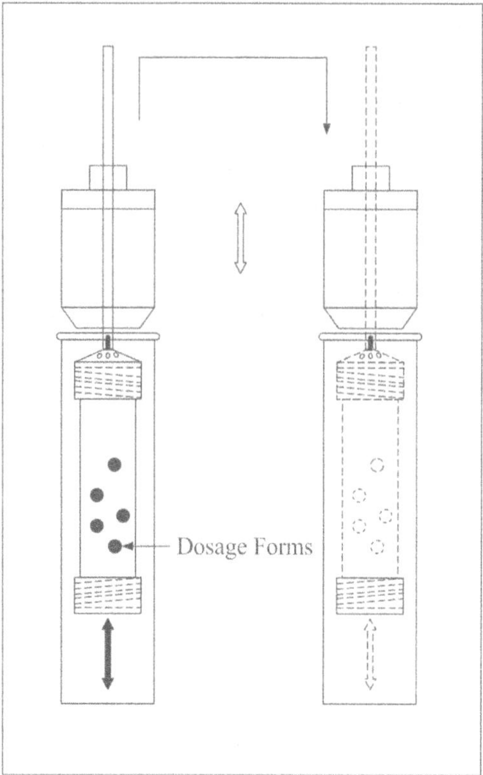

Fig. 5 USP Dissolution Testing apparatus (Reciprocating Cylinder)

3. Apparatus III can be especially useful in cases where one or more pH/buffer changes are required in the dissolution testing procedure, for example, enteric-coated/sustained release dosage forms, and also offers the advantages of mimicking the changes in physiochemical conditions and extraordinarily strong mechanical forces experienced by the drug products in the mouth or at certain locations in the GI tract, such as the pylorus and the ileocecal valve.

4. Apparatus III is currently commercially available with seven columns of six rows, each row consisting of a set of cylindrical, flat bottomed glass outer vessels, a set of reciprob.

5. The screens are made of suitable materials designed to fit the top and bottom of the reciprocating cylinders. Operation involves the agitation, in dips per minute (dpm), of the inner tube within the outer tube. On the upstroke, the bottom tube in the inner tubes moves

upward to contact the product and on the down stroke the product leaves the mesh and floats freely within the inner tube. Thus, the mechanics subject the product being tested to a moving medium.

6. The USP Apparatus III is considered as the first line apparatus in product development of controlled-release preparations, because of its usefulness and convenience in exposing products to mechanical as well as a variety of physicochemical conditions which may influence the release of products in the Gastro Intestinal (GI) tract.

7. The particular advantage of this apparatus is the technically easy and problem free use of test solutions with different pH values for each time interval. It also avoids cone formation for disintegrating (immediate release) products, which can be encountered with the USP apparatus II.

8. Ease of sampling, automation, and pH change during the test run, made this as the method of choice.

9. An additional advantage of apparatus III includes the feasibility of drug-release testing of chewable tablets. Chewable tablets for human use do not contain disintegrants, so they need to undergo physiological grinding (i.e., chewing) prior to dissolution.

10. 5dpm (dips per min) in apparatus III is equivalent to 50 rpm in Apparatus II.

USP APPARATUS IV (FLOW-THROUGH-CELL)

PRINCIPLE AND DESIGN

1. The flow-through-cell apparatus consists of a reservoir for the dissolution medium and a pump that force dissolution medium through the cell holding the test sample. Flow rate ranges from 4 to 16 ml/min. six samples are tested during the dissolution testing. And the medium is maintained at 37°C.

2. Apparatus IV may be used for modified-release dosage forms that contain active ingredients having very limited solubility.

3. There are many variations of this method. Essentially, the sample is held in a fixed position while the dissolution medium is pumped through the sample holder. Thus dissolving the drug, Laminar flow of

the medium is achieved by using a pulse less pump. Peristaltic or centrifugal pumps are not recommended.

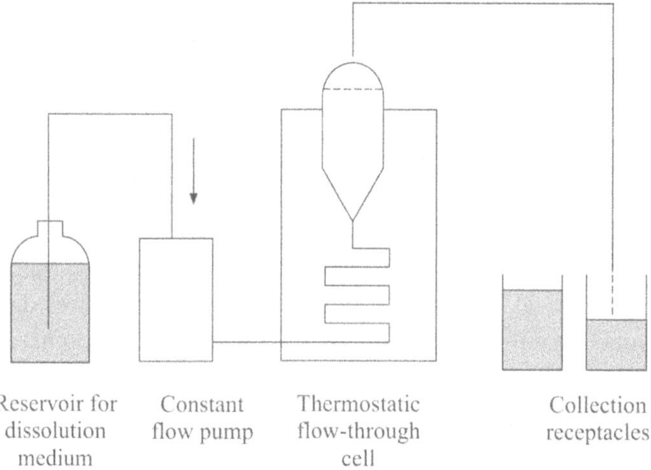

Fig 6 Continuous flow through Cell

4. The flow rate is usually maintained between 4 to 16 ml/min. The dissolution medium may be fresh or recirculated. In the case of fresh medium, the dissolution rate at any moment may be obtained, whereas in the official paddle or basket method, cumulative dissolution rates are monitored.

5. A major advantage of the flow-through method is the easy maintenance of a sink condition for dissolution. A large volume of dissolution medium may also be used, and the mode of operation is easily adapted to automated equipment.

6. The fixed solvent volume of maximal 2000 ml is kept at a temperature of 37° C. The flow through method uses an unlimited amount of solvent. There are a number of advantages compared to the apparatus I and II.

7. Sink conditions can easily be reached with Apparatus IV. Also pH changes during the test are easily performed. The media change is performed by switching a valve from one medium to another medium. As the cell volume is only about 10 ml and a typical flow rate is 16 ml/min it only requires about one minute for a complete pH change. Sampling in stirrer methods often leads to problems.

8. The introduction of the sampling probe can change the hydrodynamics and therefore the dissolution conditions. In addition, the sampling position must always be at the same point to guarantee reproducibility. In the flow through method there are no problems related to sampling.

9. Neither manual nor automated manipulations are necessary. The sample solution is automatically filtered upon leaving the cell and can be analyzed directly or after fractioning without interference of the dissolution process.

DISSOLUTION EFFICIENCY

Dissolution efficiency is defined as the area under the dissolution curve up to a certain time 't', expressed as a percentage of the area under the rectangle described by 100% dissolution in the same time.

$$DE = \left(\int_{0}^{t} y.dt \right) \times \frac{100}{Y_{100}}.t$$

DE can assume a range of values depending on the time intervals chosen for interpretation. This should be preferably greater than t_{90}% value of the formulation. Constant intervals are chosen for comparison. For example the index DE^{30} would relate to the dissolution of the drug from a particular formulation after 30min and could only be compared with the DE^{30} of other formulation.

SUITABILITY OF TEST DEVICE

Individually test one tablet (disintegrating & non disintegrating each) of the USP dissolution calibrator, according to operating conditions specified. The apparatus is suitable if the results obtained are with in the acceptance range stated in the certificate for that calibrator in the apparatus tested.

Disintegrating Type: Prednisone Calibrating Tablets

USP Prednisone Tablets *RS – current lot P0E203*

(10 mg nominal prednisone content per tablet)

- disintegrating type
- paddle and basket, 50 rpm
- 500 ml deaerated water, 37°C

- quantity of prednisone released after 30 minutes is determined specified ranges

    Lot P0E203:   Apparatus 1:   47-82 %

                            Apparatus 2:   37-70 %

Non Disintegrating Type: Salicylic Acid Calibrating Tablets

USP Salicylic acid Tablets *RS – current lot Q0D200*

(300 mg nominal salicylic acid content per tablet)

- nondisintegrating type

- paddle and basket, 100 rpm

- 900 ml deaerated phosphate buffer, 37°C

- quantity of salicylic acid, released after 30 minutes is determined specified ranges

    Lot Q_0 D200:   Apparatus 1:   23-30 %

                         Apparatus 2:   17-25 %

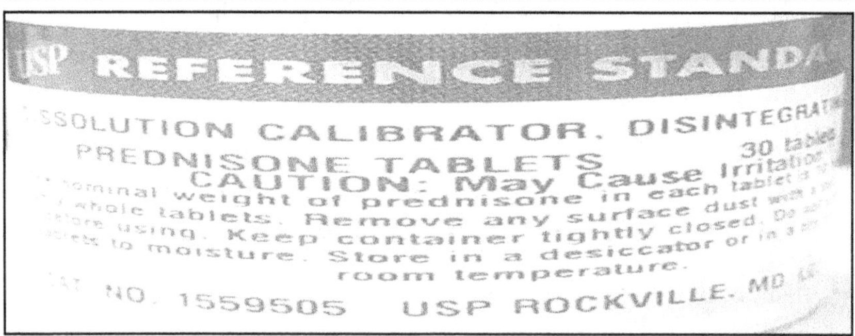

Fig. 7 USP Reference Standard Tablets

Table 2 Calculation of % Drug Release

Time (Min)	Abs	D.F	Concentration (μg.mL)	Amount (mg)	Cumulative Amount	% Drug Release
5	Ab_5	DF_5	$C5 = (Ab_5 \times DF_5)\backslash$ Slope	$A_5 = C_5 \times 0.9$	$CA_5 = A_5$	$\%DR_5 = (CA_5 \ast 100)/D$
10	Ab_{10}	DF_{10}	$C_{10} = (Ab_5 \times DF_{10})\backslash$ Slope	$A_{10} = C_{10} \times 0.9$	$CA_{10} = A_{10} + (5C_5/1000)$	$\%DR_{10} = (CA_{10} \ast 100)/D$
15	Ab_{15}	DF_{15}	$C_{15} = (Ab_5 \times DF_{15})\backslash$ Slope	$A_{15} = C_{15} \times 0.9$	$CA_{15} = A_{15} + (5C_5/1000 + 5C_{10}/1000)$	$\%DR_{15} = (CA_{15} \ast 100)/D$
20	Ab_{20}	DF_{20}	$C_{20} = (Ab_5 \times DF_{20})\backslash$ Slope	$A_{20} = C_{20} \times 0.9$	$CA_{20} = A_{20} + (5C_5/1000 + 5C_{10}/1000 + 5C_{15}/1000)$	$\%DR_{20} = (CA_{20} \ast 100)/D$
25	$Ab2_5$	DF_{25}	$C_{25} = (Ab_5 \times DF_{25})\backslash$ Slope	$A_{25} = C_{25} \times 0.9$	$CA_{25} = A_{25} + (5C_5/1000 + 5C_{10}/1000 + 5C_{15}/1000 + 5C_{20}/1000)$	$\%DR_{25} = (CA_{25} \ast 100)/D$
30	Ab_{30}	DF_{30}	$C_{30} = (Ab_5 \times DF_{30})\backslash$ Slope	$A_{30} = C_{30} \times 0.9$	$CA_{30} = A_{30} + (5C_5/1000 + 5C_{10}/1000 + 5C_{15}/1000 + 5C_{20}/1000 + 5C_{25}/1000)$	$\%DR_{30} = (CA_{30} \ast 100)/D$

DIFFUSION

Introduction

Diffusion is defined as a process of mass transfer of individual molecules of a substance. In general, molecules are in random brownian motion in matter. They move more readily from a higher concentration to a lower concentration, i.e., concentration gradient.

The diffusion of drugs through barrier is important. This barrier may be synthetic (polymeric) or natural membrane. The term barrier is applied to the region or regions that offer resistance to the passage of materials. The term membrane is normally used to a film separating the phases. The material that undergoes the transport is known as diffusant or permeant or penetrant. The material transport across the film may be by passive or facilitated diffusion.

The membrane may have pores, channels or may be nonporous. Molecular diffusion through nonporous media depends on dissolution of the permeant in the bulk membrane. Movement through pores and channels involves passage through solvent filled pores in the membrane. This process is influenced by the size of the molecules and the diameter of the pores.

Applications of Diffusion

1. The release of drugs from dosage form is diffusion controlled. Such dosage forms are available in the market as sustained and controlled release products.

2. Molecular weight of polymers can be estimated from diffusion process.

3. The transport of drugs (absorption) from gastrointestinal tract, skin, etc., can be understood and predicted from the principles of diffusion.

4. The diffusion of drugs into tissues and their excretion through kidneys can be anticipated through diffusion studies.

5. The processes such as dialysis, micro filtration, ultra filtration (in the purification of colloids), haemodialysis, osmosis etc., use the principles of diffusion. These experiments can be used as *in vitro* models for drug protein binding studies.

Methods and Procedures

For the diffusion studies, two compartment cells are used. These are:

a. Horizontal transport cell

b. Vertical transport cell

In general, horizontal cells (Viles-Chein transport cells) are used to study the skin permeation of drugs and used as *in vitro* models for drug absorption. Vertical two compartment cell is used for diffusion of gases and liquids. The diffusion of drugs from ointments, transdermal drug delivery systems can be studied using these cells.

The diffusion cells are made of glass, plexiglas, pyrex or plastic. The cells are transparent so that stirring speed (mechanism) can be visualized. These are easy to assemble or clean. The cells are jacketed and thermostated in order to maintain the temperature.

Barriers are used to separate the compartments. These are as follows.

Natural origin: Isolated biological membranes are obtained from animals.

(a) Stratum corneum (stripped skin of the forearm) is used to study percutaneous absorption.

(b) Buccal mucosa (obtained from calf buccal cavity) is used to study buccal absorption from oral cavity

(c) Human skin (obtained from autopsy) and cadaver skin (obtained from dead bodies) are used to study transdermal drug absorption.

Synthetic origin: These are used in the study of transport as *in vitro* models. Some of them are:

(a) Visking dialysis membrane is used to study protein binding and determination of molecular weight.

(b) Polyvinyl chloride is used in controlling the diffusion of drugs from controlled release systems.

(c) Polyvinyl acetate is used as rate controlling membrane in the design of controlled drug delivery systems.

General method of study of diffusion

Normally, the diffusant in the form of a solution is placed in upper compartment of the cell (donor compartment). Solvent alone or vehicle (diffusion medium) is placed in lower chamber (receptor compartment). Stirring rate and temperature are closely monitored at constant value.

In diffusion studies, the solution in the receptor compartment is constantly removed and replaced by fresh solvent to maintain constant volume. This procedure to certain ensures the sink conditions, as the concentration of diffusant in the receptor compartment at any point of time will be low.

During diffusion process, the diffusant penetrate through the membrane and reach the solvent. Hence, the concentration of diffusant in the upper compartment decreases continuously and in the lower compartment increases. Actually, after sufficient period of time, equilibrium state reaches, wherein the concentration of diffusant remain same in both sides. But in case of sink conditions, the equilibrium will not be attained. Thus steady state diffusion is achieved.

The study of diffusion is done by using kinetic method. Periodically samples are withdrawn from the receptor compartment and the concentration of diffusant is analyzed by a suitable analytical method. The kinetic data is plotted by taking time on X-axis, and % drug diffused on Y-axis.

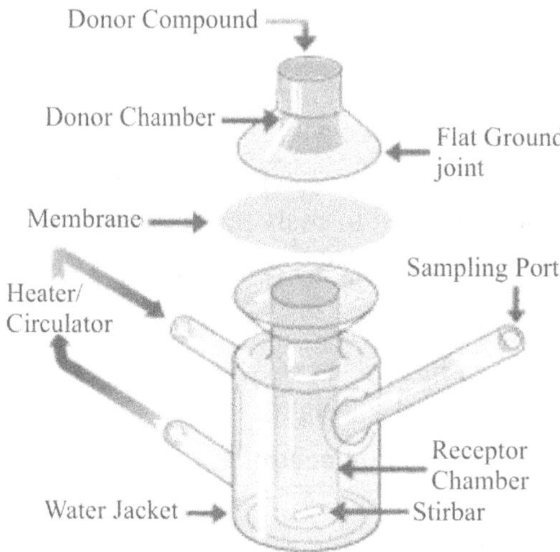

Fig 1 Horizontal Diffusion cell

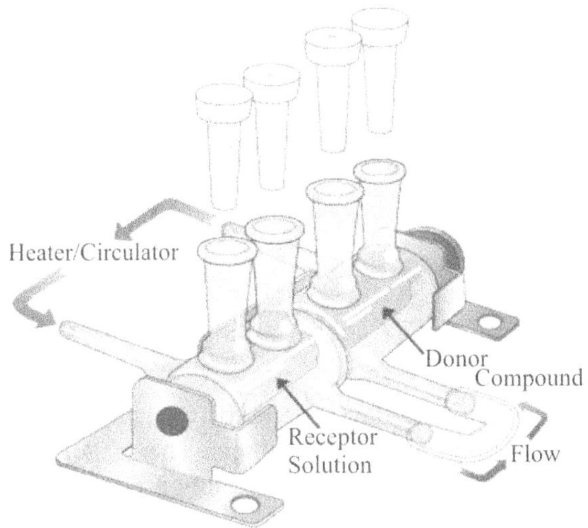

Fig 2 Vertical (Franz) Diffusion cell

KINETIC MODELS OF DRUG DISSOLUTION

The mathematical models are used to evaluate the kinetics and mechanism of drug release from the tablets. The model that best fits the release data is selected based on the correlation coefficient (r^2) value in various models. The model that gives high 'r^2' value is considered as the best fit of the release data.

INTERPRETATION OF DISSOLUTION DATA

Mathematical Dissolution Models

1. Zero order release model
2. First order release model
3. Hixson-crowell release model
4. Higuchi release model
5. Korsmeyer-peppas release model

1. Zero Order Release Equation

$$Q_t = Q_0 - K_0 t$$

Where $\quad$ Q_0 - Initial amount of drug

Q_t - Cumulative amount of drug remained to be released at time "t"

K_0 - Zero order release constant

t - Time in hours

- It describes the systems where the drug release rate is independent of its concentration of the dissolved substance

- A graph is plotted between the time on X-axis and cumulative percentage of drug release on Y-axis, and it gives a straight line with negative slope.

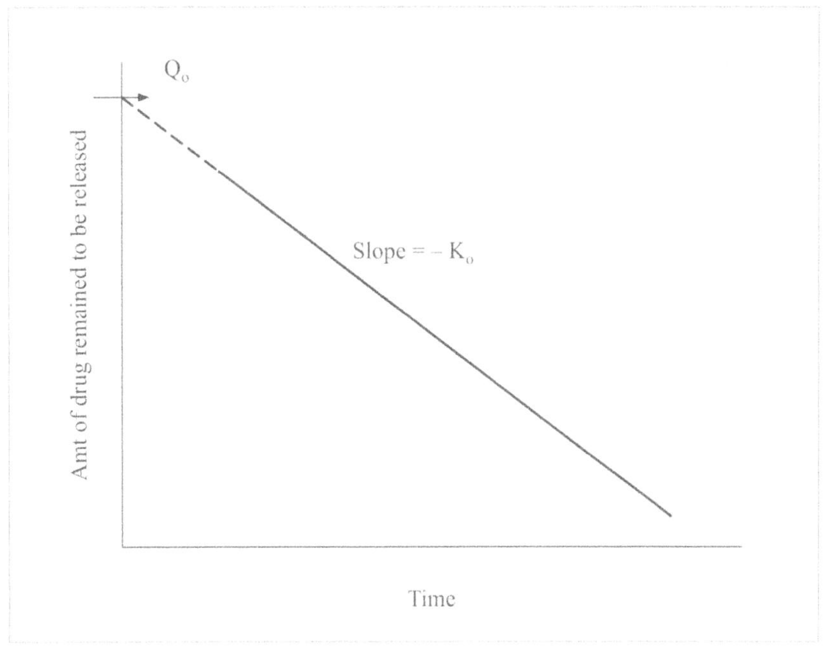

Fig. 1 Plot of Zero order drug release.

2. First Order Release Equation

$$\log Q_t = \log Q_0 - K_t / 2.303$$

Where

Q_0 - initial amount of drug

Q_t - Amount of drug remaining to be released at time "t"

K - first order release constant

t - time in hours

- It describes the systems where the drug release rate is dependent of its concentration of the dissolved substance

- A graph is plotted between the time on X-axis and log amt of drug remaining to be released on Y-axis, and it gives a straight line with negative slope.

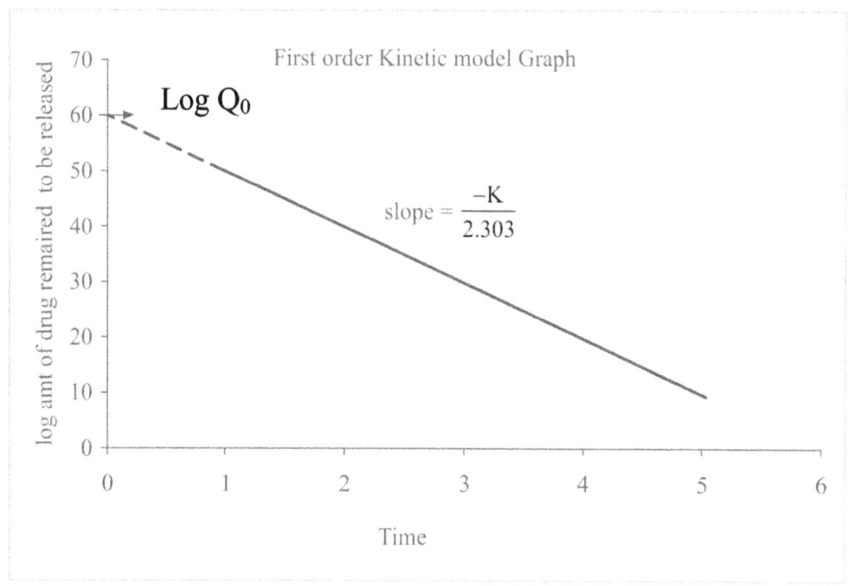

Fig. 2 Plot of First order drug release.

3. Hixson-Crowell Release Equation:

$$\sqrt[3]{Q_0} - \sqrt[3]{Q_t} = K_{HC}t$$

Where

Q_0 - Initial amount of drug

Q_t - Amount of drug remained to be released at time "t"

K_{HC} - Hixson crowell release constant

t   - time in hours

- It describes the drug release by dissolution and with the change in surface area and diameter of the particles or tablets

- A linear plot of the cube root of the initial concentration minus the cube root of the percent remaining versus time in hours for the dissolution data in accordance with the hixon crowells model.

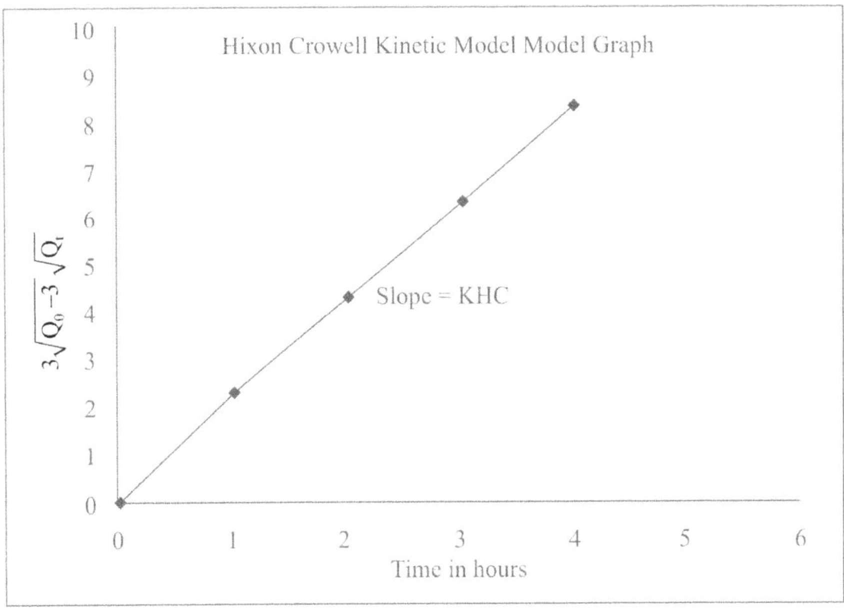

Fig. 3 Plot of Hixson-Crowell model of drug release.

4. Higuchi Release Equation

$$Q_t = K_H\, t^{1/2}$$

where

Q - Cumulative amount of drug release at time "t"

K_H - Higuchi constant

t   - Time in hours

- Higuchi equation suggests that the drug release is by diffusion.

- A graph is plotted between the square root of time taken on x-axis and the cumulative amount of drug release on y-axis and it gives a straight line.

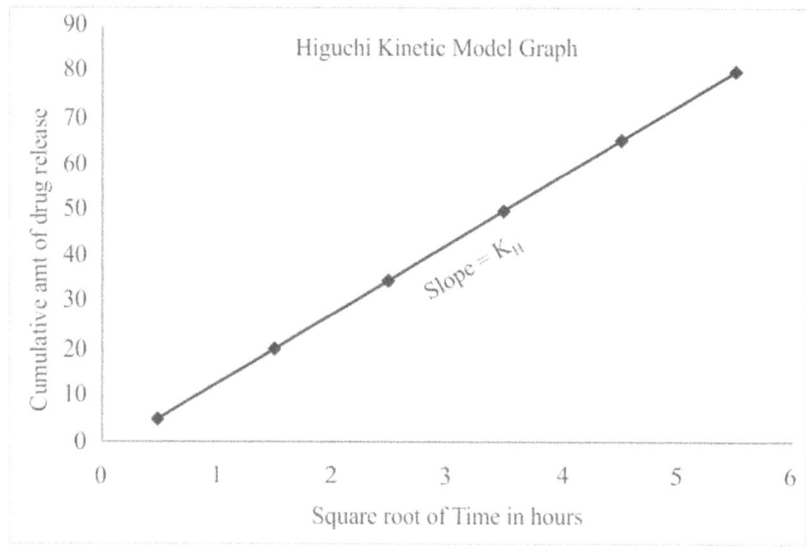

Fig. 4 Plot of Higuchi model of drug release.

5. Korsmeyer-Peppas Equation

$$\text{Log}(M_t/M) = \log K_m + n \log t$$

where

F	-	Fraction of drug released at time 't'
M_t	-	Amount of drug released at time 't'
M	-	Total amount of drug in dosage form
K_m	-	Kinetic constant
n	-	Diffusion or release exponent
t	-	Time in hours

- 'n' is estimated from linear regression of log(Mt/M) versus log t
- If 'n' = 0.45 indicates fickian distribution
- 0.45<n< 0.89 indicates anomalous diffusion or non-fickian distribution
- If 'n' = 0.89 and above indicates case 2 relaxation or super case transport 2
- Anomalous diffusion or non fickian diffusion refers to combination of both diffusion and erosion controlled rate release.

- Case 2 relaxation or super case transport 2 refers to the erosion of the polymeric chain.
- A graph is plotted by taking log time on X axis, and log M_t/M (log fraction dissolved) on Y axis and it gives a straight line.

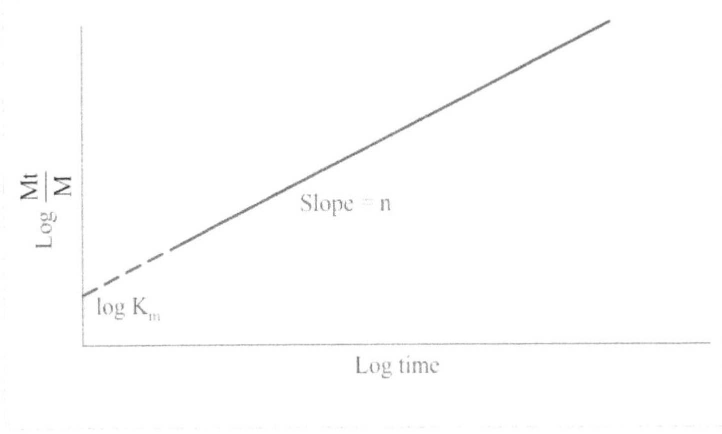

Fig. 5 Plot of Korsmeyer Peppas model of drug release.

APPENDIX 6

STATISTICAL TECHNIQUES

Introduction

1. Most of the pharmaceutical investigations involve experimental studies with an aim to compare a sample statistic with the population parameter or statistics of sample from two or more populations with specific and distinct characteristics.

2. In experimental pharmaceutics, very often we come across two-group experimental design wherein one of the group is "treated" and the other is the "control".

3. Statistics of "treated" and "control" groups are compared to infer about the respective populations.

4. In all the comparisons, the aim is to assess whether there is significant difference between a sample statistic and the corresponding population parameter or between two parameters or between more than two parameters

5. Difference may be due to "error" that occurs naturally.

6. **Hypothesis:** The hypothesis may be that the sample mean is lesser than the population mean, or the mean of treated group is greater than the mean of the control group or the means of more than two groups are not the same. These hypotheses may be shown symbolically as follows

$$H: \overline{X} < \mu$$

$$H: \mu_1 > \mu_2$$

$$H: \mu_1 \neq \mu_2 \neq \mu_3 \neq \mu_4$$

7. **Null Hypothesis:** The null form of the hypothesis (H) is called the null –hypothesis (H₀), which means that there is no significant difference between the means of the two groups. The null hypothesis of the above hypothesis represented as followos.

$$\mathbf{H_0}: \overline{X} - \mu = 0$$

or $\mathbf{H_o}: \overline{X} = \mu$

or $\mathbf{H_o}:\ \mu_1 = \mu_2$

or $\mathbf{H_o}:\ \mu_1 = \mu_2 = \mu_3 = \mu_4$

8. Verbally, the H_o states that there is no significant difference between sample mean and population mean, or between means of two populations, or between means of more than two populations.

9. **Level of Significance (LS):** It is an arbitrarily selected point in the probability scale, below which the probability is considered low, and equal to or above which the probability is considered high. Conventionally 0.05 (5%) or 0.01 (1%) of level of significance is used in biostatistics

10. **Degrees of freedom (DF):** The DF of **a** distribution is defined as the number of variates that can be entered in that distribution before the values of the remainder of the variates are fixed by the necessity to produce a certain total. Usually the degrees of freedom of any distribution is assumed as n-1 (n is total number of variables).

STUDENT'S t-TEST

1. **Matched Pair Data Analysis:** One of the experimental designs in pharmacy is to assign the same subjects both for "control" and "experimental" treatments. For example, if an investigator wants to evaluate the efficacy of a new drug formulation in reducing the blood glucose levels in man, he/ she can have a sample of 10 persons who are willing to undergo the experiment. The usual procedure is to divide the sample of 10 persons into two groups and administer the placebo and the drug to each group. In the matched pair design, all the ten persons are given, first, the placebo treatment and their blood samples are analysed for blood glucose level. Next, after the expiry of sufficient time, the same persons are given the drug, and their blood samples are analysed for blood glucose level. Thus, each subject yields a pair of data, which can be analysed using the t-test to assess significance of the mean difference.

Method

(a) Same subject yields pairs of data ex: (i). values obtained before and after treatment; (ii) values obtained after control treatment and after experimental treatment; (iii) values obtained at two different periods –now and after a gap of a day, a month, a year etc.,

(b) Significance of the mean difference (D*) is tested using t-test

(c) H_0: D* – μ_D = 0; n – 1 degrees of freedom (n = pairs of data); sampling distribution of mean difference (D*'s) with a population mean of μ_D = 0

(d) Computation:

    (i) D = difference between n pairs of values

    (ii) $\sum D$

    (iii) Mean difference, D = $\sum D/n$

    (iv) $\sum(D - D*)^2$

(v) Sandard deviation, SD = $\sqrt{(\sum(D - D*)^2/n)}$

(vi) Standard error of mean difference, S_D = SD/$\sqrt{(n-1)}$

(e) t= D- μ_D/S_D

(f) Note table "t" at specific LS and DF

(g) Decision: If calculated t > table 't', reject H_0

(h) Inference: Based on the decision, the given H is discussed

Example of problem

A pharmaceutical company develops a drug, which it claims to increase hemoglobin content in aged people. The hemoglobin content (g/100 ml) of 10 subjects is measured before and after administration of the drug. On the basis of the following data determine whether the company's claim is valid.

Subject	1	2	3	4	5	6	7	8	9	10
Before	10	9	11	12	8	7	12	18	10	9
After	12	11	13	14	9	10	12	14	11	12

Step 1: H_0: D* – μ_D = 0; LS = 0.05; DF = 10 – 1 = 9

Step 2: Computation of SD

Before	After	D	D – D*	$(D - D*)^2$
10	12	2	0	2
9	11	2	0	0
11	13	2	0	0
12	14	2	0	0
8	9	1	– 1	1

Table Contd...

Before	After	D	D – D*	(D – D*)^2
7	10	3	1	1
12	12	0	– 2	4
10	14	4	2	4
10	11	1	– 1	1
9	12	3	1	1
		20		12

D* = ΣD / n = 20/10 = 2 g/100 mg/100 ml

SD = $\sqrt{12/10}$ = $\sqrt{1.2}$ = 1.1 mg/100ml

Step 3: assumption of sampling distribution of D* with a mean of μ_D = 0 and SE computed as

SE of mean difference = SD/$\sqrt{}$ (n – 1) = 1.1/$\sqrt{}$ (10 – 1) =1.1/3 = 0.37

Step 4: Location of observed mean difference in the sampling distribution in terms of 't as

$$t = (D*- \mu_D)/SE = 2/0.37 = 5.41$$

Step 5: Decision about the H_0: D* – μ_D = 0

Table't' at 0.05 LS, and 9 DF = 1.833

The calculated t (5.42) > table't'; Reject H_0

Step 6: The sample mean difference is significant. The drug is effective in increasing the hemoglobin content in aged people. The claim of the company is valid

2. **Comparison of means of two groups:** A more common design of experiment is to assign different subjects to two groups. It is assumed that the two groups are samples from two different populations such as "control population" and "experimental population". Using student's t-test we can assume sampling distribution of difference between means, compute the SE of difference between means, locate the observed difference between means in the sampling distribution in terms of the t value. The calculated t-value is compared with the table t at specified LS and DF, a decision is made about H_0 and inference is drawn about the population difference between means.

Method

1. Data: Group 1: n_1, X^*_1, S_1 and Group 2: n_2, X^*_2, S_2

2. H_0: $\mu_1 - \mu_2 = 0$ (no significant difference between the means of the two population from which the sample n_1 and n_2 were obtained, respectively)

3. Sampling distribution of differences between means. Standard error of difference between means of two uncorrelated groups is obtained using pooled variance ($S_p{}^2$)

$$S_p{}^2 = \frac{\left(n_1 S_1{}^2 + n_2 S_2{}^2\right)}{\left(n_1 + n_2\right)}$$

$$SE = \sqrt{\frac{\left(s_p\right)^2}{n_1 - 1} + \frac{\left(s_p\right)^2}{n_2 - 1}}$$

4. Calculation of t-value as, $t = (X^*_1 - X^*_2)/SE$

5. Table t at specified LS and $n_1 + n_2 - 2$ degrees of freedom

6. Decision: If calculated t > table t, reject H_0

7. Inference: based on the decision the given H is discussed

Example

Dissolution study was conducted to two different brands of same drug formulation, and the amount of drug release within first five min from six tablets of each brand are given in the following table. Can we say the dissolution from the brand 1 is higher than brand 2?

| Amount of drug release | Brand 1 | 6.2 | 5.7 | 6.5 | 6.0 | 6.3 | 5.8 |
| | Brand 2 | 5.6 | 5.9 | 5.6 | 5.7 | 5.8 | 5.7 |

Step 1:

Brand 1	Brand 2
$n_1 = 6$	$n_2 = 6$
$X^*_1 = 6.08$	$X^*_2 = 5.716$
$S_1 = 0.279$	$S_2 = 0.116$

Step 2: H_0: $\mu_1 - \mu_2 = 0$; LS = 0.05; DF = 6 + 6 − 2 = 10

Step 3: Assumption of a sampling distribution between means, with a mean $\mu_1 - \mu_2 = 0$ and SE of difference between means computed as follows

$$S_p^2 = (n_1S_1^2 + n_2S_2^2)/(n_1+n_2) = 0.045$$

$$SE = \sqrt{0.018} = 0.134$$

Step 4: Location of the observed difference between means in the sampling distribution in terms of t,

$$t = 2.72$$

Step 5: Decision about the H_0: Table $t_{0.05LS \text{ and } 10DF} = 1.812$

Since the calculated 't' > the table 't', H_0: $\mu_1 - \mu_2 = 0$ is rejected. There is significant difference between the means of two brands

Step 6: Inference: The amount of drug release of brand 1 is significantly higher than brand 2.

ANALYSIS OF VARIANCE (ANOVA)

Introduction

1. Use of t-test is rather difficult in situations where we have to compare the parameters of more than two populations, for the obvious reason of increasing number of tests we will have to perform to compare each pair of means in all possible combinations. Further, the probability of error would become enormous, proportional to the number of tests.

2. The ANOVA is the appropriate statistical technique to be used in situations where we have to compare more than two groups.

3. If we want to compare more than two groups with $n_1, n_2, n_3......n_k$ samples and $X^*_1, X^*_2, X^*_3......X^*_k$ means, these groups might be experimental groups with different treatments or might be samples from populations which are different in some specific feature. The observed differences between these groups will consist of two components, viz., a natural variation (error) and variation due to treatment or any other factor.

4. In ANOVA, the two components of the observed difference are separated, estimated and compared. The variation due to "treatment" is expected to occur between groups and therefore is referred to as "between variance". The natural variation would occur within each of the groups and therefore referred to as the "within variance". The variations from the two sources, "between" and "within" together is called the "total variance"

5. If "within" variability is greater than the "between" variability, it would mean that the difference between groups is not significant. On

the other hand, if the "between" variability is greater than the "within" variability, it would suggest a significant difference between groups.

Method:

ONE WAY ANOVA

Step1: Correction Factor (CF) = $(\sum X)^2/N$

Step 2: Total sum of squares $(SS_{total}) = \sum X^2 - CF$

Step 3: Between sum of squares $(SS_{between}) = (\sum X_a)^2/n_a + (\sum X_b)^2/n_b + \ldots\ldots + (\sum X_k)^2/n_k - CF$

Step 4: Within sum of squares or Error sum of squares $(SS_{within}) = SS_{total} - SS_{between}$

Step 5: Construction of ANOVA table

Sources of variation	Degrees of freedom	Sum of Squares (SS)	Mean squares (MS)	F Ratio
Between	k–1	$SS_{between}$	$MS_{between} = SS_{between}/(k-1)$	$F = MS_{between}/MS_{within}$
Within	N–k	SS_{within}	$MS_{within} = SS_{within}/(N-k)$	
Total	N–1	SS_{total}	$MS_{total} = SS_{total}/N-1$	

Step 6: Null Hypothesis: H_0: $\mu_1 = \mu_2 = \mu_3 = \mu_k$

The meaning of the null hypothesis is that there is no significant difference among the means of the populations.

Step 7: If the F Value is equal to or less than 1, it is obvious that "within" group variance is equal to or greater than "between" variance and therefore, there is no significant difference between the means of populations.

Step 8: If the F value is greater than 1, then we will have to check the significance of the observed F with the table values of F at specific levels of significance and appropriate degrees of freedom. If the calculated F is greater than table F, we reject the null hypothesis

Step 9: On the basis of the decision taken, we discuss the given hypothesis

Example

The following data represent the AUC values of four different formulations in human volunteers. Analyze these data for significant difference among the bioavailability of four formulations?

Subject	AUC (μg.hr/ml)			
	F1	F2	F3	F4
A	4	8	5	1
B	5	7	7	4
C	1	9	8	1
D	3	6	6	3
E	2	10	9	1

Step 1: Correction factor: $CF = (100)^2/20 = 500$

Step 2: $SS_{total} = 668 - 500 = 168$

Step 3: $SS_{between} = (15)^2/5 + (40)^2/5 + (35)^2/5 + (10)^2/5 - 500 = 130$

Step 4: $SS_{within} = 168 - 130 = 38$

Step 5:

Sources of variation	Degrees of freedom	Sum of Squares (SS)	Mean squares (MS)	F Ratio
Between	$4 - 1 = 3$	$SS_{between} = 130$	$MS_{between} = 130/3 = 43.33$	$F =$
Within	$19 - 3 = 16$	$SS_{within} = 38$	$MS_{within} = 38/16 = 2.375$	$43.33/2.375$
Total	$20 - 1 = 19$	$SS_{total} = 168$	--	$= 18.24$

Step 6: Null Hypothesis: $H_0: \mu_1 = \mu_2 = \mu_3 = \mu_4$

Step 7: The F Value is not equal to or not less than 1, so it is obvious that "within" group variance is lesser than "between" variance

Step 8: The F value is greater than 1, and then we will have to check the significance of the observed F with the table values of F at specific levels of significance and appropriate degrees of freedom.

Table value of F with 3 and 16 degrees of freedom at 0.05 LS = 3.24

Since the calculated F (18.24) > table F (3.24), we reject the H_0. This means, the bioavailability of four formulations are not same. (P<0.05)

Step 9: There is significant difference among four formulations in terms of bioavailability

TWO WAY (MULTIPLE) ANOVA

Step 1: Correction Factor (CF) $= (\sum X)^2/N$

Step 2: Total sum of squares (SS$_{total}$) $= \sum X^2 - CF$

Step 3: Between order sum of squares

$SS_{order} = [(\sum X_{order1})^2 + (\sum X_{order2})^2 + \ldots\ldots + (\sum X_{order\,k})]/n_{subjects} - CF$

Step 4: Between formulation sum of squares

$SS_{formulation} = [[(\sum X_{form1})^2 + (\sum X_{formu2})^2 + \ldots\ldots + (\sum X_{form\,k})]/n_{subjects} - CF$

Step 5: Between Subject sum of squares

$SS_{subject} = [[(\sum X_{sub1})^2 + (\sum X_{subj2})^2 + \ldots\ldots + (\sum X_{sub\,k})]/n_{formulations} - CF$

Step 6: Error sum of squares

$SS_{error} = SS_{total} - SS_{order} - SS_{formulation} - SS_{subject}$

Step 7: Construction of ANOVA table

Sources of variation	Degrees of Freedom	Sum of Squares (SS)	Mean Squares (MS)	F Ratio
Between order	DF_O = Number of orders -1	SS_{order}	$MS_{order} =$ SS_{order}/DF_O	$F_{(Order,\ Error)} =$ MS_{order}/MS_{error}
Between formulation	DF_F = Number of formulations -1	$SS_{formulations}$	$MS_{formulation} =$ $SS_{formulation}/DF_F$	$F_{(Formulation,\ Error)} =$ $MS_{Formulation}/MS_{error}$
Between subjects	DF_S = Number of Subjects -1	$SS_{subjects}$	$MS_{Subjects} =$ $SS_{Subjects}/DF_S$	$F_{(Subject,\ Error)} =$ $MS_{Subjects}/MS_{Error}$
Error	$DF_E = DF_T - DF_O - DF_F - DF_S$	SS_{error}	$MS_{error} =$ SS_{error}/DF_E	---
Total	$DF_T = N - 1$	SS_{total}		

Step 8: Null Hypothesis: H_0: $\mu_1 = \mu_2 = \mu_3 = \mu_k$

The meaning of the null hypothesis is that there is no significant difference among the means of the populations.

Step 9: If the F Value of any variable is equal to or less than 1, it is obvious that error variance is equal to or greater than "between" variance and therefore, there is no significant difference between the means of populations.

Step 10: If the F value any variable is greater than 1, then we will have to check the significance of the observed F with the table values of F at specific levels of significance and appropriate degrees of freedom. If the calculated F is greater than table F, we reject the null hypothesis

Step 11: On the basis of the decision taken, we discuss the given hypothesis

Example

A bioequivalence study was conducted by CRO, for optimized formulation of tablet (Test formulations) with the marketed formulation of same drug (Reference product). They have followed the two way cross over design. Data obtained is given in the following table. Find out whether the all formulations are bioequivalent to that of reference product or not by using Multiple ANOVA technique?

Reference Product Code: A

Test Products Codes: B

Subjects	AUC Values (mcg.hr/ml)			
	Period I		Period II	
1	Test	23	Reference	36
2		25		35
3		23		37
4		29		38
5		24		39
6		22		30
7	Reference	31	Test	26
8		33		27
9		35		28
10		37		24
11		36		26
12		39		24

Step 1: Correction factor:

$CF = (\sum X)^2/N = (23+25+.....36+39+.....+36+35+.....26+24)^2/24 = (727)^2/24 = =22022.04$

Step 2: Total sum of squares

$SS_{total} =$
$(529+625+529+841+576+484+961+1089+1225+1369+1296+1521+1296 +1225+1369+1444+1521+900+676+729+784+576+676+576) - 22022.04 =22817-22022.04 =794.96$

Step 3: Between order sum of squares

$SS_{order} = [(357)^2 + (370)^2/12] -22022.04= [(127449+136900)/12]- 22022.04 =7.043$

[Note: $\sum X_{order1} = 357$; $\sum X_{order2} = 370$]

Step 4: Between formulation sum of squares

$SS_{formulation} = [(301)^2 + (426)^2/12] -22022.04 = [(90601+181476)/12] - 22022.04 = 651.043$

[Note: $\sum X_{test\ formulation} = 301$; $\sum X_{reference\ formulation} = 426$]

Step 5: Between Subjects sum of squares

$SS_{Subject} = [[(59)^2 + (60)^2 + (60)^2 + (67)^2 + (63)^2 + (52)^2 + (57)^2 + (60)^2 + (63)^2 + (61)^2 + (62)^2 + (63)^2]/2] - 22022.04$

$SS_{Subject} = (3481 + 3600 + 3600 + 4489 + 3969 + 2704 + 3249 + 3600 + 3969 + 3721 + 3844 + 3969)/2 - 22022.04 = 22097.5 - 22022.04 = 75.46$

Step 6: Error sum of squares = $\mathbf{SS_{Error}}$ = 794.96 −7.043 − 651.043 − 75.46 = 61.414

Step 7: Construction of ANOVA table.

Sources of variation	Degrees of Freedom	Sum of Squares (SS)	Mean Squares (MS)	F Ratio
Between order	$DF_0 = 2 - 1 = 1$	7.043	$MS_{order} = 7.043$	$F_{(Order,\ Error)} = 7.043 / 6.14 = 1.14$
Between formulation	$DF_F = 2 - 1 = 1$	651.043	$MS_{formulation} = 651.043$	$F_{(Formulation,\ Error)} = 651.04 / 6.14 = 106.03$
Between subjects	$DF_S = 12 - 1 = 11$	75.46	$MS_{Subjects} = 6.86$	$F_{(Subject,\ Error)} = 6.86 / 6.14 = 1.11$
Error	$DF_E = 23 - 1 - 1 - 11 = 10$	61.414	$MS_{error} = 6.14$	---
Total	$DF_T = 24 - 1 = 23$	794.9		

Step 8: Null Hypothesis: H_0: $\mu_1 = \mu_2$

The meaning of the null hypothesis is that there is no significant difference among the means of the populations.

Step 9:

The 'F' Value of any variable is not equal to or less than 1, it is obvious that error variance is lesser than "between" variance and therefore, there is significant difference between the means of populations.

Step 10:

Order Variance:

F value of order variable is greater than 1, and then we will have to check the significance of the observed F with the table values of F at specific levels of significance and appropriate degrees of freedom.

The table value at 1, 10 degrees of freedom is 4.96. And the calculated F is **lesser than** table F, so there is no significant effect of order of administration on bioavailability

Formulation Variance:

F value of formulation variable is greater than 1, and then we will have to check the significance of the observed F with the table values of F at specific levels of significance and appropriate degrees of freedom.

The table value at 1, 10 degrees of freedom is 4.96. And the calculated F is **greater than** table F, so there is significant difference between formulations and hence not bioequivalent and hypothesis is rejected.

Subject Variance:

F value of subject variable is greater than 1, and then we will have to check the significance of the observed F with the table values of F at specific levels of significance and appropriate degrees of freedom.

The table value at 11, 10 degrees of freedom is 2.86. And the calculated F is **lesser than** table F, so there is no significant effect of subject on drug bioavailability.

Step 11: On the basis of the results obtained it can be concluded that the bioavailability of test formulation is not equivalent to reference formulation. There was a significant difference between formulations and there was no difference between order and subjects.

APPENDIX 7

BIOAVAILABILITY AND BIOEQUIVALENCE STUDIES

PURPOSE OF BIOAVAILABILITY STUDIES

Bioavailability studies are usually performed for both approved active drugs and therapeutic moieties not yet approved for marketing by the FDA. In approving a drug product for marketing, the FDA ensures that the drug product is safe and effective for its labeled indications for use. To ensure the standards of identity, strength, quality, and purity, the FDA requires bioavailability/pharmacokinetic studies and, where necessary, bioequivalence studies for all drug products. Data from *in-vivo* bioavailability studies are important to establish recommended dosage regimens and to support drug labeling. *In-vivo* bioavailability studies are also performed for new formulations of active drug ingredients or therapeutic moieties that have full NDA approval and are approved for marketing. The purpose of these studies is to determine the bioavailability and to characterize the pharmacokinetics of the new formulation, new dosage form, or new salt or ester relative to a reference formulation. In summary, clinical studies are useful in determining the safety and efficacy of drug products. Bioavailability studies are used to define the effect of changes in the physicochemical properties of the drug substance and the effect of the drug product (dosage form) on the pharmacokinetics of the drug. Bioequivalence studies are used to compare the bioavailability of the same drug (same salt or ester) from various drug products. Bioavailability and bioequivalence can also be considered as performance measures of the drug product *in vivo*. If the drug products are bioequivalent and therapeutically equivalent (as defined above), then the clinical efficacy and the safety profile of these drug products are assumed to be similar and may be substituted for each other.

112

METHODS FOR ASSESSING BIOAVAILABILITY

(I) Indirect/ Pharmacokinetic Methods:

Plasma drug concentration

1. Time for peak plasma (blood) concentration (t max)
2. Peak plasma drug concentration (C max)
3. Area under the plasma drug concentration–time curve (AUC)

Urinary drug excretion

1. Cumulative amount of drug excreted in the urine (Xu)
2. Rate of drug excretion in the urine (dXu/dt)
3. Time for maximum urinary excretion (t)

(II)Direct/ Pharmacodynamic Methods:

Acute pharmacodynamic effect

1. Maximum pharmacodynamic effect (E max)
2. Time for maximum pharmacodynamic effect
3. Area under the pharmacodynamic effect–time curve
4. Onset time for pharmacodynamic effect

Clinical observations

- Well-controlled clinical trials

In-vitro studies

- Drug dissolution

BIOAVAILABILITY STUDY PROTOCOL

I.   **Title**
  A.   Principal investigator (study director)
  B.   Project/protocol number and date

II.   **Study objective**

III.   **Study design**
  A.   Design
  B.   Drug products
    1. Test product(s)
    2. Reference product
  C.   Dosage regimen
  D.   Sample collection schedule
  E.   Housing/confinement

    F.   Fasting/meals schedule

    G.   Analytical methods

IV. Study population

    A.   Subjects

    B.   Subject selection

        1. Medical history

        2. Physical examination

        3. Laboratory tests

    C.   Inclusion/exclusion criteria

        1. Inclusion criteria

        2. Exclusion criteria

    D.   Restrictions/prohibitions

V. Clinical procedures

    A.   Dosage and drug administration

    B.   Biological sampling schedule and handling procedures

    C.   Activity of subjects

VI. Ethical considerations

    A.   Basic principles

    B.   Institutional review board

    C.   Informed consent

    D.   Indications for subject withdrawal

    E.   Adverse reactions and emergency procedures

VII. Facilities

VIII.Data analysis

    A.   Analytical validation procedure

    B.   Statistical treatment of data

IX. Drug accountability

    X. Appendix

BIOAVAILABILITY STUDY DESIGNS

Three different studies may be required for solid oral dosage forms, including (1) a fasting study, (2) a food intervention study, and/or (3) a multiple-dose (steady-state) study. Proper study design and statistical evolution are important considerations for the determination of bioequivalence.

Fasting Study

Bioequivalence studies are usually evaluated by a single-dose, two-period, two-treatment, two-sequence, open-label, randomized crossover design comparing equal doses of the test and reference products in fasted, adult, healthy subjects (Male And Female).

Food Intervention Study

Co-administration of food with an oral drug product may affect the bioavailability of the drug. Food intervention or food effect studies are generally conducted using meal conditions that are expected to provide the greatest effects on GI physiology so that systemic drug availability is maximally affected.

Multiple-Dose (Steady-State) Study

In a few cases, a multiple-dose, steady-state, randomized, two-treatment, two-way crossover study comparing equal doses of the test and reference products may be performed in adult, healthy subjects.

Latin-Square Crossover Design for a Bioequivalence Study of Three Drug Products in Six Human Volunteers

Subject	Drug Product		
	Study Period 1	Study Period 2	Study Period 3
1	A	B	C
2	B	C	A
3	C	A	B
4	A	C	B
5	C	B	A
6	B	A	C

Latin-Square Crossover Design for a Bioequivalency Study of Four Drug Products in 16 Human Volunteers

Subject	Drug Product			
	Study Period 1	Study Period 2	Study Period 3	Study Period 4
1	A	B	C	D
2	B	C	D	A
3	C	D	A	B
4	D	A	B	C
5	A	B	D	C
6	B	D	C	A

Table *contd...*

Subject	Drug Product			
	Study Period 1	Study Period 2	Study Period 3	Study Period 4
7	D	C	A	B
8	C	A	B	D
9	A	C	B	D
10	C	B	D	A
11	B	D	A	C
12	D	A	C	B
13	A	C	D	B
14	C	D	B	A
15	D	B	A	C
16	B	A	C	D

Period refers to the time period in which a study is performed. A two-period study is a study that is performed on two different days (time periods) separated by a washout period during which most of the drug is eliminated from the body–generally about 10 elimination half-lives.

APPENDIX 8

PHARMACOKINETICS

INTRODUCTION TO PHARMACOKINETICS
ONE COMPARTMENT OPEN MODEL-IV
BOLUS-PLASMA-PARENT DRUG

Theory

In a pharmacokinetic analysis of the data, the living system (human body) is assumed to consist of a number of interconnected compartments. Compartment can be defined as a single kinetically homogeneous unit. A compartment consists of group of tissues which behaves uniformly with respect to the drug movement. The open indicates that the bioavailability and elimination are unidirectional and the drug is eliminated from the central compartment i.e., blood.

One compartment model is particularly useful for drugs which rapidly distribute between plasma and other body fluids and tissues upon entry into the systemic circulation. However, this model does not mean that drug concentration in each tissue is the same at any given point of time. The one compartment open model assumes that any changes that occur in the plasma levels of the drug reflect proportional changes in the tissue drug levels. The following assumptions are made in deriving mathematical equations to describe one compartment open model

1. The drug absorption always follows first order rate kinetics and its rate constant Ka is apparent first order absorption rate constant

2. Any changes that occur in the plasma levels of the drug reflect proportional changes in the tissue drug levels.

3. Once the drug enters the systemic circulation, it rapidly distributes to other body fluids and tissue, and a dynamic equilibrium is achieved instantaneously between the drug in the blood and other tissues.

4. Elimination of the drug from the body follows an apparent first order kinetics and its rate constant K, is known as an apparent first order rate constant.

117

The schematic representation of drug movement in the body in this case is shown below

$$X_0 \longrightarrow \boxed{X = V_d . C} \xrightarrow{\ K\ }$$

Where

X_0 = Dose of drug injected

X = Amount of drug present in body at any time 't'

V_d = Apparent volume of distribution of drug

C = Concentration of drug in central compartment at any time 't'

K = apparent overall first order elimination rate constant

DERIVATION OF FIRST ORDER KINETICS

The rate of decrease of the amount of the drug in the body is depends on the amount of the drug present in the body at any given time following I.V. bolus. Thus we can write as follows,

$$\frac{dX}{dt} \alpha X \qquad\qquad .....(1)$$

Where dX/dt is the change in amount of the drug with respect to change in time

$$\frac{dX}{dt} = -KX \qquad\qquad .....(2)$$

Where 'K' is a first order rate constant, negative sign indicates that the drug is being lost from the body.

To obtain the total amount of drug lost from the body within the given period of time after injection, eq. 2 must be integrated after separating the variables

$$\int_0^t \frac{dX}{X} = \int_0^t -Kdt \qquad\qquad .....(3)$$

$$\left|\ln X\right|_0^t = -K\left|t\right|_0^t \qquad\qquad .....(4)$$

$$\ln X - \ln X_0 = -K(t-0) \qquad\qquad .....(5)$$

$$\ln X = \ln X_0 - Kt \qquad\qquad .....(6)$$

By applying logarithms

$$\log X = \log X_0 - \frac{Kt}{2.303} \qquad .....(7)$$

The equation 7 can be written in exponential form,

$$X = X_0 e^{-kt} \qquad .....(8)$$

Equations 7 to 8 denote the amount of drug in the body with respect to time. To describe the plasma drug concentration with respect to time the above equations can be written in concentration terms by utilizing apparent volume of distribution (V_d).

$$i.e\ X = V_d.\ C$$

Substituting the values of X in equation 7, we get

$$\log C = \log C_0 - \frac{Kt}{2.303}$$

Where

C_0 = concentration of drug in plasma at time, t = 0

C = concentration of drug in plasma at any time 't'

The above equation is in the form of straight line $Y = mX + C$

Where   Y = log C;

X = t;

Slope = m = -K/2.303;

Intercept = C = log C_0;

So on Cartesian graph paper the following graph is obtained

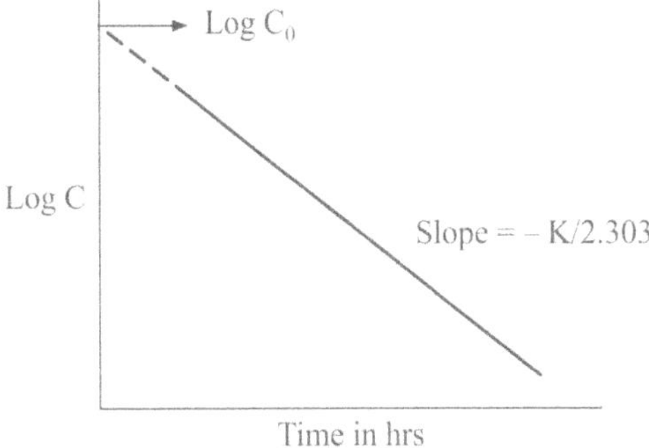

Fig. 1 A plot of log concentration of drug versus time following IV Bolus.

Semi-logarithmic plot of plasma concentration vs. time can be also plotted. Semi-logarthmic paper is available with one, two, three or more cycles per sheet, each cycle representing a 10 fold increase in numbers, or single log 10 units.

The starting value of Y-axis should never be zero. If the starting value is 1, the next cycle starts with 10 and next with 100. The intercept can be obtained by extending the line to time zero.

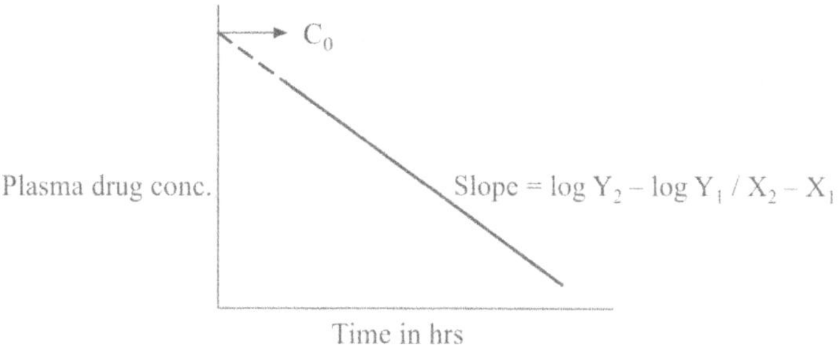

Fig. 2 Semi-logarithmic plot of plasma drug concentration

versus time following IV Bolus.

DERIVATION OF PHARMACOKINETIC PARAMETERS

1. **Elimination rate constant K**: An overall apparent first order rate constant is the sum of the rate constants of all the processes involved in elimination of the drug which is denoted as 'K'

   The value of K can be obtained from the slope. The rate constant K has the dimensions of reciprocal of time, since log C is dimensionless.

   $$K = - (\text{Slope}) \times 2.303$$

2. **Biological Half-life $t_{1/2}$:** The time required for the concentration to fall to a half of its initial value.

   $$\log C = \log C_0 - \frac{Kt}{2.303}$$

   By rearranging the above equation,

   $$\log \frac{C_0}{C} = \frac{Kt}{2.303} \quad \text{When } C_0/C = 2, \text{ then } t = t_{1/2}$$

   $$\log 2 = \frac{Kt_{1/2}}{2.303}$$

$$0.3 = \frac{Kt_{1/2}}{2.303}$$

$$Kt_{1/2} = 0.3 \times 2.303 = 0.693$$

$$K = \frac{0.693}{t_{1/2}} \quad \text{or} \quad t_{1/2} = \frac{0.693}{K}$$

3. **Hypothetical Volume of Distribution (V_d):** The hypothetical volume of body fluids within which a drug is uniformly distributed is known as the volume of distribution. It does not refer to any physiological fluid volume. It is calculated simply by dividing the I.V. dose by drug concentration in plasma at t=0, by C_0. Hence, the value of V_d only represents a theoretical volume in which the drug is assumed to be uniformly distributed.

V_d = I.V dose (X_0) / Initial concentration (C_0)

Lipid soluble drugs have more binding affinity to tissue proteins than the plasma proteins thus have a large V_d, and are more concentrated in extra vascular compartment. Highly soluble, poorly penetrating drugs are bound lightly to tissue proteins and bound highly to plasma proteins and thus have a smaller V_d. Drugs which bind to tissues will have a large Vd, because of low C_0 values. For each drug V_d is constant. In certain pathological cases the apparent V_d for the drug may be altered.

4. **Area Under the Curve AUC:** AUC is an important parameter often estimated by several methods. It is expressed in µg h/mL. It is the total integrated area under the plasma concentration versus time profile. The most common method for estimating the area is the use of Trapezoidal rule. The curve is divided into trapeziums based on data and the sum of areas of all trapeziums gives Area Under the Curve up to the last sampling AUC_{0-t}.

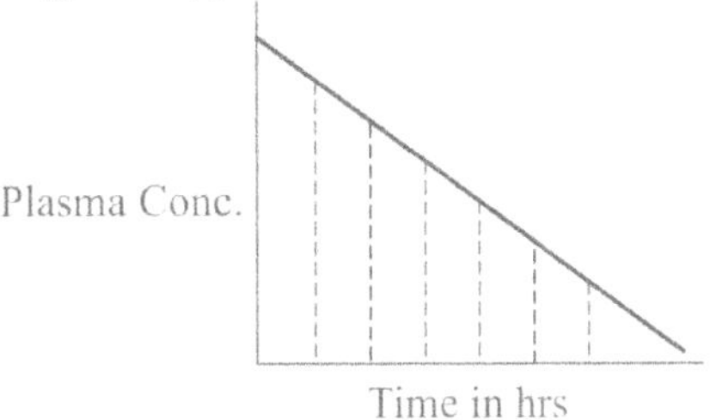

Fig. 4 Plot of plasma concentration versus time

$AUC_{0-t} = 0.5\ (C_0 + C_1)\ (t_1 - t_0) + 0.5\ (C_1 + C_2)\ (t_2 - t_1) + \text{----} + 0.5\ (C_{n-1} + C_n)\ (t_n - t_{n-1})$

The remaining Area under the Curve from the last point to $t=\infty$ is calculated by integration method

$$AUC_{t-\infty} = C^* / K$$

Where C^* is the concentration of the drug at the last time point, t^*

The total Area Under the Curve from $t = 0$ to $t = \infty$ is given by

$$AUC_{0-\infty} = AUC_{0-t} + AUC_{t-\infty}$$

Note: Another method to calculate $AUC_{0-\infty}$ is based on integration method

$$AUC_{0-\infty} = C_0 / K \text{ where } C_0 \text{ is initial conc. at } t = 0$$

Clearance Cl: Clearance is defined as the volume of body fluid from which the drug is cleared in unit time and is expressed as mL/min or L/h. Total body clearance is the sum of all the clearances that contribute to drug elimination

$$Cl_t = Cl_{metab} + Cl_{renal}, \text{ etc.}$$

The rate of elimination of a drug from the body is directly proportional to the plasma concentration.

Rate of elimination $dX/dt\ \alpha\ C_p$ where C_p = plasma concentration

Or $\qquad dX/dt = Cl_t\ C_p$

The proportionality constant Cl_t is known as total body clearance. Total amount of drug eliminated from the body in infinite time is obtained by integrating the above equation with respect to time between $t=0$ and $t=\infty$

$$\int_0^\alpha dX = Cl_t \int_0^\alpha C_p dt$$

Total amount eliminated

$$= Cl_t \left[AUC\right]_0^\alpha \text{ Since } \int_0^\alpha C_p dt = \left[AUC\right]_0^\alpha$$

$\therefore$ Total body clearance, Cl_t = Total amount of drug eliminated / $\left[AUC\right]_0^\alpha$

In the case of IV bolus injection, total drug eliminated is equal to the administered dose (X_0).

$$Cl_t = X_0 \text{ (IV dose)} / [AUC]_0^\alpha$$

But $X_0 = V_d\, C_0$ and $[AUC]_0^\alpha = C_0 / K$ substituting these values in above equation

$$Cl_t = \frac{V_d . C_0}{C_0 / K} = V_d . K$$

5. Area under the Mean Curve AUMC

AUMC is the total integrated area under (plasma concentration X time) versus (time) curve which is often estimated by several methods. It is expressed in $\mu g\, h^2/mL$. The most common method for estimating the area is the use of Trapezoidal rule. The curve is divided into trapeziums based on data and the sum of areas of all trapeziums gives Area Under the Curve up to the last sampling $AUMC_{0-t}$.

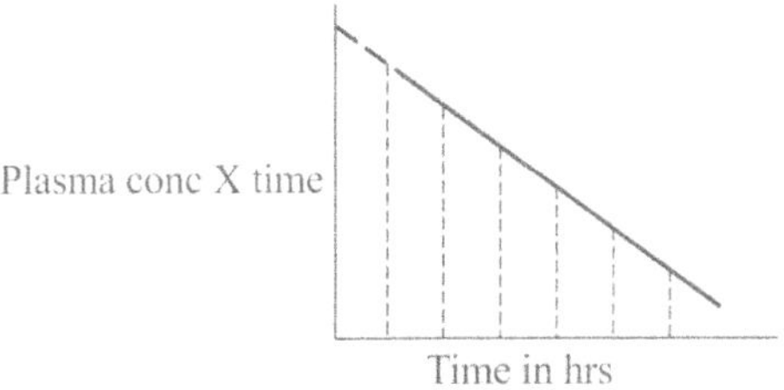

Fig. 5 Plot of plasma concentration x time versus time.

$AUMC_{0-t} = 0.5\ (C_0 t_0 + C_1 t_1)\ (t_1 - t_0) + 0.5\ (C_1 t_1 + C_2 t_2)\ (t_2 - t_1) + \text{----} + 0.5\ (C_{n-1} t_{n-1} + C_n t_n)\ (t_n - t_{n-1})$

The remaining Area under the Curve from the last point to $t = \infty$ is calculated by integration method

$$AUMC_{t-\infty} = [C^* t^* / K] + [C^*/K^2]$$

Where C^* is the concentration of the drug at the last time point, t^*

The total Area Under the Curve from $t = 0$ to $t = \infty$ is given by

$$AUMC_{0-\infty} = AUMC_{0-t} + AUMC_{t-\infty}$$

Note: Another method to calculate $AUMC_{0-\infty}$ is based on integration method

$$AUMC_{0-\infty} = C_0 / K^2 \text{ where } C_0 \text{ is initial conc. at } t = 0$$

Formulae

1. Intercept $= C_0$ (µg/mL or ng/mL or g/L)

2. Slope $= [\log (Y_2) - \log (Y_1)]/(t_2 - t_1)$ or $[\log (C_2) - \log (C_1)]/(t_2 - t_1)$

3. Overall Elimination Rate Constant $K(\ h^{-1}) = (-\text{Slope}) \times 2.303$

4. Elimination Half – Life $t_{1/2}$ (h) $= 0.693/K$

5. Apparent Volume of Distribution V_d (L) $= X_0 / C_0$

6. Area Under the Curve (AUC_0^{∞}) (µg.h/mL)$= AUC_0^{t} + AUC_t^{\infty}$

7. AUC_0^{t} (Trapezoidal Rule) (µg.h/mL) $= [(C_0 + C_1)/2] (t_1-t_0) + [(C_1+ C_2)/2] (t_2-t_1) + ---+ [(C_{n-1}+ C_n)/2] (t_n-t_{n-1})$

8. AUC_t^{∞} (Integration Method) (µg.h/mL) $= C^* / K$

9. AUC_0^{∞} (Integration Method) (µg.h/mL) $= C_0 / K$

10. Area Under the Mean Curve $AUMC_0^{\infty}$ (µg.h^2/mL) $= AUMC_0^{t} + AUMC_t^{\infty}$

11. $AUMC_0^{t}$ (Trapezoidal Rule) (µg.h^2/mL) $= [(C_0 t_0 + C_1 t_1)/2] (t_1-t_0) + [(C_1 t_1+C_2 t_2) /2](t_2-t_1)+----+ [(C_{n-1} t_{n-1} + C_n t_n)/2](t_n- t_{n-1})$

12. $AUMC_t^{\infty}$ (µg.h^2/mL) $= [C^* t^*/K] + C^*/K^2$

13. $AUMC_0^{\infty}$ (Integration Method) (µg.h^2/mL) $= C_0 / K^2$

14. Mean Residence Time (H) $= AUMC_0^{\infty}/ AUC_0^{\infty} = 1/K$

15. Total clearance CL_T (L/h) $= \text{Dose} / AUC_0^{\infty} = V_d . K$

DERIVATION OF PHARMACOKINETIC PARAMETERS – ONE COMPARTMENT OPEN MODEL - IV BOLUS – UNCHANGED DRUG IN URINE

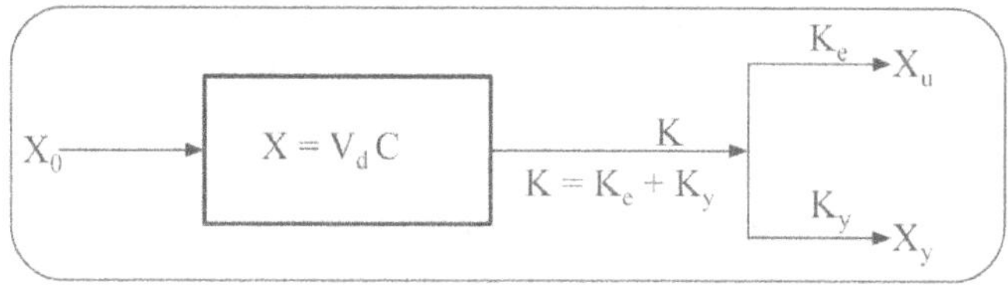

Schematic Representation

X_0 - Dose Administered (mg)

X - Amount of Drug present in the compartment at any time 't'

V_d - Apparent Volume of distribution (mL or L)

C   -   Plasma Concentration (μg/mL or ng/mL)

K   -   Overall Apparent Elimination Rate Constant (h^{-1})

K_e -   Excretion rate constant through renal pathway (h^{-1})

K_y -   Excretion rate constant through non renal pathway (h^{-1})

X_u -   Cumulative Amount of drug that ultimately excreted through renal pathway (mg)

X_y -   Cumulative Amount of drug that ultimately excreted through non renal pathway (mg)

I. EXCRETION RATE METHOD

The rate of disappearance of the unchanged drug in urine is directly proportional to the amount of the drug in the body as urinary excretion of a drug follows the first order kinetics. The urinary excretion rate of the unchanged drug dXu / dt can be defined as,

$$\frac{dX_u}{dt}\,\alpha X$$

$$\frac{dX_u}{dt} = K_e X$$

X is the amount of the drug in the body at any time t. But as per plasma model of IV bolus, the unchanged drug in blood is given as

$$X = X_0 e^{-kt}$$

Substituting the value of X in above equation

$$\frac{dX_u}{dt} = K_e X_0 e^{-kt}$$

Applying logarithms to the equation, we get

Log $(dX_u)/dt = \log [K_e X_0 e^{-Kt}]$

Log $(dX_u)/dt = \log K_e X_0 + \log e^{-Kt}$

$$\log\frac{dX_u}{dt} = \log K_e X_0 - \frac{Kt}{2.303}$$

The term dXu/dt is instant rate of excretion. The excretion rates are obtained experimentally by determining the amount of the drug excreted in a given period of time. The mean excretion rate in the given period of time is $\Delta Xu/\Delta t$ which closely approximates dXu/dt at the mid point of urine collection time interval (t^1).

So, above equation can be written as

$$\log \frac{\Delta X_u}{\Delta t} = \log K_e X_0 - \frac{Kt^1}{2.303}$$

The above equation is in the form of straight line $Y = mX + C$

Where $Y = \log \Delta X_u/\Delta t$;

$$X = t^1;$$

Slope = m = $- K/2.303$;

Intercept = C = $\log K_e X_0$.

Therefore, a plot of log $\Delta Xu/\Delta t$ versus t^1 yields a straight line with a slope of $- K/2.303$.

This is the same slope as is obtained from semilogarithmic plot of plasma concentration of drug versus time. Thus, the elimination rate constant, K of a drug can be obtained from either plasma concentration of drug versus time data or urinary excretion data.

Note: It must be remembered that the slope of the log excretion rate versus t^1 is a function of the elimination rate constant, K and not of the urinary rate constant, Ke. The intercept is equal to log KeX₀.

Calculation of Pharmacokinetic parameters by Excretion rate method in different cases of urine data

Case I: Data provided contain time and rate of excretion of drug

Urine data obtained following an I.V. Bolus dose is processed as following

Time (h)	Δ Xu/ Δ t (mg/h)	t^1 (h) = $(t_n + t_{n-1})/2$
---	----	-----

The average excretion rate ($\Delta Xu/\Delta t$) taken on Y-axis of semi log graph and t^1 (mid point of urine collection) on X-axis gives a straight line with a slope of $-K/2.303$ as shown in below figure.

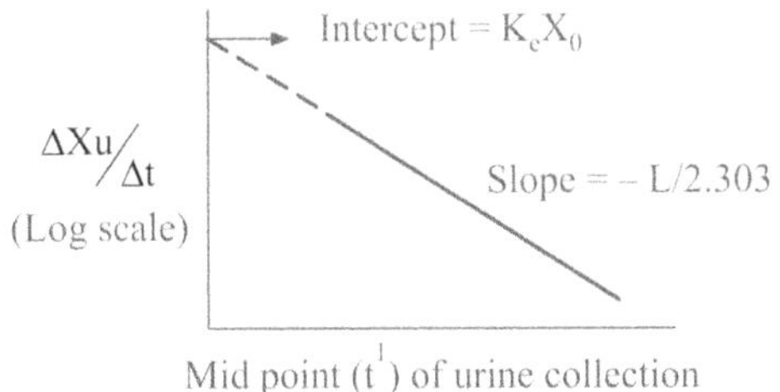

Fig. 5 Plot of Average rate of drug excretion versus midpoint of time interval

Case II: Data provided contain time and urine volume

The urine data given is first processed as following

Time (h)	Urine volume (mL)	Concentration Of drug (µg/mL)	ΔX_u (mg) [Concentration x Volume]	Δt (h) $(t_n - t_{n-1})$	$\Delta X_u / \Delta t$ (mg/h)	t^1 (h) $(t_n + t_{n-1})/2$
-----	-----	-----	-----	-----	-----	-----

Then obtained average excretion rate ($\Delta Xu / \Delta t$) taken on Y-axis of semi log graph and t^1 (midpoint of urine collection) on X-axis gives a straight line with a slope of $-K/2.303$ same as shown in above figure

Case III: Data provided contain time and cumulative amount of drug excreted in urine

The urine data given is first processed as following

Time (h)	Cumulative amount of drug in urine (mg)	dX_u or ΔXu (mg)	dt or Δt (h)	$\Delta Xu / \Delta t$ (mg/h)	t^1 (h) $(t_n + t_{n-1})/2$
-----	-----	-----	-----	-----	-----

Then obtained average excretion rate ($\Delta Xu / \Delta t$) taken on Y-axis of semi log graph and t^1 (midpoint of urine collection) on X-axis gives a straight line with a slope of $-K/2.303$ same as shown in above figure

Parameters can be determined

1. *Over all elimination rate constant*, K can be calculated from the slope.

Slope = $- K/2.303$

K = Slope × 2.303

2. ***Biological half-life*** of the drug can be calculated using K, value.

$$t_{1/2} = 0.693 / K$$

3. ***Urinary excretion rate constant***, $\mathbf{K_e}$: the intercept obtained by extending the straight line is equal to $K_e X_0$. Since the dose administered is known, K_e can be calculated.

4. ***Fraction of dose excreted unchanged***, $\mathbf{fe} = K_e / K$

Formulae at glance:

1. Intercept $= K_e X_0$ (mg/h)

2. Slope $= \dfrac{\log\left(Y_2\right) - \log\left(Y_1\right)}{X_2 - X_1}$

3. Overall Elimination Rate Constant $K(h^{-1}) = (-\text{Slope}) \times 2.303$

4. Elimination Half – Life $t_{1/2}$ (h) $= 0.693/K$

5. Renal Excretion Rate Constant $(K_e)(h^{-1}) = \text{Intercept}/X_0$

6. Non Renal Excretion Rate Constant $(K_y)(h^{-1}) = K - K_e$

7. Renal Clearance CL_R (L/h) $= V_d . K_e$

8. Non Renal Clearance CL_{NR} (L/h) $= V_d . K_y$

9. Total Clearance CL_T (L/h) $= CL_R + CL_{NR}$

10. Total Clearance CL_T (L/h) $= V_d K$

11. Fraction unchanged dose that ultimately excreted through renal pathway $f_e = K_e/K$

12. Amount unchanged dose that ultimately excreted through renal pathway $X_u = f_e X_0$

II. SIGMA MINUS METHOD

An alternative method other method used to analyze urinary excretion data is Sigma-minus method. In this method the assumption of $dXu / dt \sim \Delta X_u / \Delta t$ is not required.

The urinary excretion rate of drug is directly proportional to the amount of the drug in body,

$$dX_u/dt \; \alpha \; X$$

$$\frac{dX_u}{dt} = K_e X$$

$X = X_0 e^{-kt}$ Substituting the value of X in above equation

$$\frac{dX_u}{dt} = K_e X_0 e^{-kt} \qquad \qquad .....(1)$$

Integrating the equation with respect to time between the limits of t=0 to t=t

$$\int_0^t dX_u = \int_0^t K_e X_0 e^{(-Kt)} dt$$

$$\left. X_u \right|_0^t = K_e X_0 \frac{\left| e^{-Kt} \right|_0^t}{-K} \qquad [\, \textstyle\int e^{2x}\, dx = e^{2x}/2]$$

$$X_u^t - X_u^0 = K_e X_0 \left| \frac{e^{-kt}}{-K} + \frac{e^0}{K} \right| \qquad \text{but, } e^0 = 1$$

X_u^t --- the cumulative amount of drug excreted into urine to time 't' and

X_u^0 ----the cumulative amount of the drug excreted in zero time $= 0$

$$X_u^t - 0 = K_e X_0 \left| \frac{e^{-kt}}{-K} + \frac{1}{K} \right|$$

$$X_u^t = \frac{K_e X_0}{K}\left(1 - e^{-Kt}\right) \qquad \qquad .....(2)$$

By integrating equation 1, between limits $t = 0$ to $t = \alpha$, the total amount of unchanged drug that will be excreted in urine with a dose of X_0 to time α can be obtained

$$\int_0^\alpha dX_u = \int_0^\alpha K_e X_0 e^{(-Kt)} dt$$

$$\left. X_u \right|_0^\alpha = K_e X_0 \frac{\left| e^{-Kt} \right|_0^\alpha}{-K}$$

$$\left. X_u \right|_0^\alpha = K_e X_0 \frac{\left| e^{-Kt} \right|_0^\alpha}{-K} \quad \text{But } e^\alpha = 0;\ e^0 = 1$$

$$X_u^\alpha = K_e X_0 \left| 0 + \frac{1}{K} \right|$$

$$X_u^\alpha = \frac{K_e X_0}{K}$$

Upon substituting X_u^α in equation 2 instead of $K_e X_0 / K$, the above equation can be written as follows,

$$X_u^t = X_u^\alpha \left(1 - e^{-Kt}\right)$$

$$X_u^{\ t} = X_u^{\ \infty} - X_u^{\ \infty} . e^{-kt}$$

Upon rearranging above equation

$$\therefore X_u^\alpha - X_u^t = X_u^\alpha e^{-Kt}$$

Applying logarithms to equation, we get

$$\log\left(X_u^\alpha - X_u^t\right) = \log X_u^\alpha - \frac{Kt}{2.303}$$

A value of X_u^t is subtracted at every time point from X_u^α and hence this method is called Sigma-minus method.

The above equation is in the form of straight line $Y = mX + C$

Where $Y = \log (X_u^{\ \infty} - X_u^{\ t})$;

$X = t$;

Slope $= m = - K/2.303$;

Intercept $= C = \log X_u^{\ \infty} = \log KeX_0/K$

Therefore, a plot of log log $(X_u^{\ \infty} - X_u^{\ t})$ versus 't' yields a straight line with a slope of $- K/2.303$. This is the same slope as is obtained from semi logarithmic plot of plasma concentration of drug versus time and excretion rate method slope. Thus, the elimination rate constant, K of a drug can be obtained from either plasma concentration of drug versus time data or urinary excretion data or sigma minus method.

***Calculation of Pharmacokinetic parameters by Sigma-Minus method* in different cases of urine data**

Case I: Data provided contain time and rate of excretion of drug

Urine data obtained following an I.V. Bolus dose is processed as following

Time (H)	dXu/dt (mg/h)			

Urine data obtained following an I.V. Bolus dose is processed as following

Time (h)	Urine volume (mL)	Conc. Of drug (µg/mL)	X_u^t (mg) Conc. x Vol	Cumulative amount	$X_u^\alpha - X_u^t$
--	--	--		-- $X_u^\alpha =$	--

The urine data obtained following IV bolus are first processed and a semi log plot of $\log\left(X_u^\alpha - X_u^t\right)$ versus t^1 (mid point of urine collection) gives a straight line with a slope of $-K/2.303$ as shown in fig.

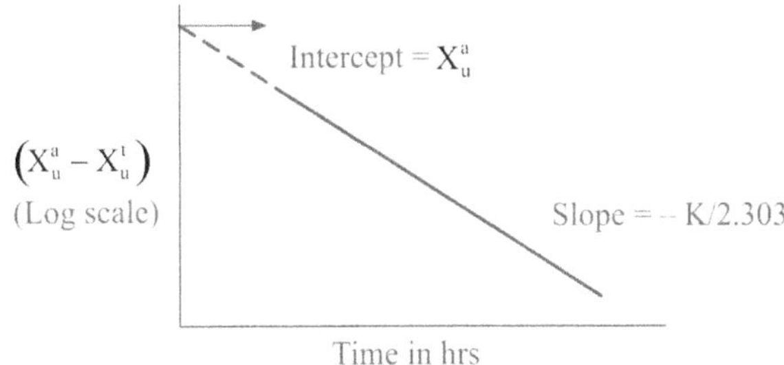

1. *Overall elimination rate constant*, K can be calculated from the slope.

Slope $= - K / 2.303$

$K = $ Slope $\times 2.303$

2. *Biological half-life* of the drug can be calculated using K, value.

$t_{1/2} = 0.693 / K$

3. *Urinary excretion rate constant*, K_e: the intercept obtained by extending the straight line is equal to X_u^α. Since the dose administered and X_u^α is known, using equation $X_u^\alpha = \dfrac{K_e X_0}{K}$, the value of K_e is calculated.

$$K_e = \frac{K X_u^\alpha}{X_0}$$

4. *Fraction of dose excreted unchanged*, f_e: $f_e = K_e / K$

Renal excretion as a fraction of total elimination

An important pharmacokinetic parameter is the fraction of the amount of drug entering the general circulation that is excreted unchanged, f_e. In case of IV bolus, f_e is a fraction of IV dose excreted in urine. When an 'f_e' value is low, urinary excretion is a minor pathway of drug elimination. Occasionally, renal excretion is the only route of elimination, in which case the values of 'f_e' is 1.0. by definition the difference $(1-f_e)$ is the fraction of the amount entering the circulation that is eliminated by extra-renal mechanisms, usually metabolism.

Formulae at glance

1. Intercept $= X_u^\infty = K_e X_0/K$ (mg)
2. Slope $= [\log (Y_2) - \log (Y_1)]/(X_2 - X_1)$
3. Overall Elimination Rate Constant $K(h^{-1}) = (-\text{Slope}) \times 2.303$
4. Elimination Half – Life $t_{1/2}$ (h) $= 0.693/K$
5. Renal Excretion Rate Constant (Ke) $(h^{-1}) = \text{Intercept}. K / X_0$
6. Non Renal Excretion Rate Constant (Ky) $(h^{-1}) = K - K_e$
7. Renal Clearance CL_R (L/h) $= V_d . K_e$
8. Non Renal Clearance CL_{NR} (L/h) $= V_d . K_y$
9. Total Clearance CL_T (L/h) $= CL_R + CL_{NR}$
10. Total Clearance CL_T (L/h) $= V_d K$
11. Fraction unchanged dose that ultimately excreted through renal pathway $f_e = K_e/K$
12. Amount unchanged dose that ultimately excreted through renal pathway $X_u = f_e X_0$

Comparison of Excretion rate method and Sigma-Minus method

Excretion rate method	Sigma-Minus method
1. Equation of this method $$\log \frac{\Delta X_u}{\Delta t} = \log K_e X_0 - \frac{Kt^1}{2.303}$$	1. Equation of this method: $$\log\left(X_u^\alpha - X_u^t\right) = \log X_u^\alpha - \frac{Kt}{2.303}$$
2. dX_u/dt is assumed to be equal to $\Delta X_u/\Delta t$	2. Such assumption is not required.
3. More no. of samples with short time intervals.	3. Less no. of samples at convenient time intervals.
4. Useful for drugs with long half-lives	4. Not suitable for drugs with long half-lives

Table *Contd....*

Excretion rate method	Sigma-Minus method
5. Any urine sample losses do not affect the method.	5. sample loss means, the whole experiment is failure
6. This method is used for multiple doses also.	6. This method is not useful for multiple dose study.
7. This method requires the collection of urine samples for 3 or 4 half-lives of the drug.	7. This method requires the collection of urine samples for 7 half-lives of the drug for an accurate assessment.
8. Intercept $= K_e X_0$ (mg/h)	8. Intercept $= X_u^\infty = K_e X_0/K$ (mg)
9. Renal Excretion Rate Constant (K_e) = Intercept $/X_0$	9. Renal Excretion Rate Constant (K_e) (h^{-1}) = Intercept $.K / X_0$

ONE COMPARTMENT OPEN MODEL- IV INFUSION- PLASMA-PARENT DRUG

Schematic Representation

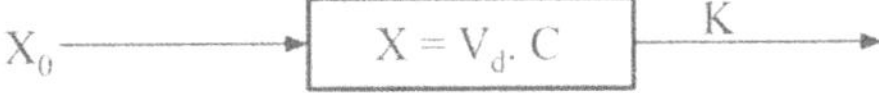

X_0 - Dose of drug administered

X - Amount of Drug present in the compartment at any time 't'

V_d - Apparent Volume of distribution (mL or L)

C - Plasma Concentration (μg/mL or ng/mL)

K - Overall Apparent Elimination Rate Constant (h^{-1})

   $K_0 = $ Zero order infusion rate const (mg/h)

General Graph

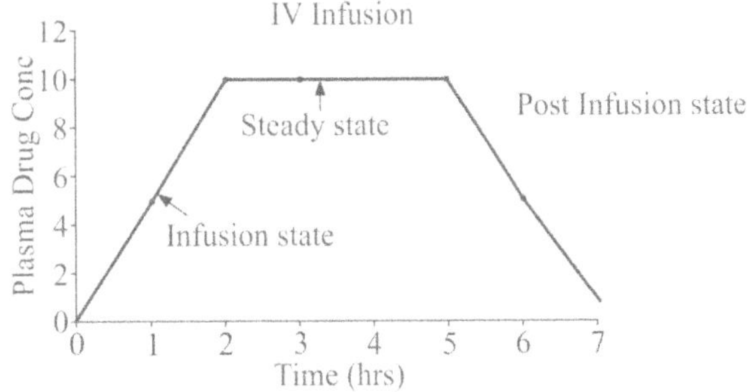

Mathematical Equations

Infusion state:

$$\text{Log } C = \log \left[(K_0/V_d K)(1 - e^{-Kt}) \right]$$

At steady state:

$$\text{Log } (C_{ss} - C) = \text{Log } C_{ss} - Kt/2.303$$

$$C_{ss} = K_0/ KV_d$$

Post Infusion state:

$$C = C_{max}. \, e^{-kt^*} \quad \text{where } t^* \text{ -- Time after infusion is stopped}$$

Two cases:

1. *Infusion is stopped after C_{ss} is achieved*

   $$\text{Log } C = \text{Log } (K_0/V_d K) - K \, t^*/2.303$$

2. *Infusion is stopped before C_{ss} is achieved (T- Total time of Infusion)*

   $$\text{Log } C = \text{Log } (K_0/V_d K)(1 - e^{-kT}) - Kt^*/2.303$$

   1. $C_{max} = (K_0/V_d K)(1 - e^{-kT})$
   2. $V_d = (K_0/K.C_{max}). \, (1 - e^{-kT})$ ---When C_{ss} not achieved
   3. $V_d = (K_0/ K.C_{ss})$ ---- When C_{ss} is achieved
   4. $Cl = \text{Dose} / AUC$ or $K_0 \, T/ AUC$
   5. $f_{ss} = 1 - e^{-kt}$
   6. $T_{95\%} = 4.32 \times t \, 1/2$

One Compartment Open Model – Extravascular – Plasma – Parent Drug

Schematic Representation

$$X_0 \longrightarrow \boxed{X = V_d . \, C} \xrightarrow{\;K\;}$$

X_0 -   Dose Administered (mg)

X   -   Amount of Drug present in the compartment at any time 't'

V_d -   Apparent Volume of distribution (mL or L)

C   -   Plasma Concentration (μg/mL or ng/mL)

K   -   Overall Apparent Elimination Rate Constant (h^{-1})

   K_a = First order absorption rate const (h^{-1})

Mathematical Equation

$$\text{Log } C = \log [K_a F X_0 / V_d (K_a - K)][e^{-kt} - e^{-Kat}]$$

Graph on Semi log Paper

X axis – Time (min / hours / days)

Y axis – Plasma parent drug concentration (µg/mL or ng/mL or mg/ mL)

1. Bell shaped curve will be obtained. By considering the last two points of curve extrapolate the curve on to Y- axis. This Line is called as **Extrapolated line**.

2. Now determine the Plasma concentrations on the extrapolated line at each time intervals. These concentrations are known as **Extrapolated Concentrations** which are denoted with **C***

3. Now substract the each plasma concentrations from extrapolated concentrations. These obtained concentrations are known as **Residual Concentrations**.

$$C_r = C^* - C$$

4. Now draw a line by pointing residual concentration values at each time period. This line is called as **Residual Line.**

Precautions to be taken while plotting the Graph:

(a) Y- Intercept of both extrapolated line and residual line should be the same value. (when there is no lag time)

(b) While extrapolating the bell shaped curve by considering last two points on to Y-axis remaining all other plasma concentrations should fall behind the extrapolated line.

(c) Draw a best fit residual line so that it should intercept the Y-axis at the same point as extrapolated line.

(d) For the determination of slope of extrapolated line consider last two points only.

(e) For the determination of slope of residual line any two points can be considered which are coming on residual line.

Formulae

1. Intercept $= (K_a F X_0)/[V_d(Ka-K)]$ (µg/mL) or $(K_a F X_0)/[V_d(K-Ka)]$ (µg/mL)

2. Slope of extrapolated line = $[\log (C_2) - \log (C_1)] / (t_2 - t_1)$

3. Slope of residual line = $[\log (C_2) - \log (C_1)] / (t_2 - t_1)$

4. Rate constant of extrapolated line (K or K_a) = $-$(slope of extrapolated line)$\times$ 2.303

5. Rate constant of residual line (K or K_a) = $-$(slope of residual line) $\times$ 2.303

6. If IV Bolus data of parent drug is available, then compare the both of these rate constant values with overall elimination rate constant value obtained with parent drug. Rate constant value which is very closer is assumed as overall elimination rate constant for parent drug (K) and other one is absorption rate constant (K_a)

7. If I.V. Bolus data of parent drug is not available, assume that $K_a > K$ and in this case final equation will be

    $\text{Log } C = \log [K_a F X_0 / V_d (K_a - K)] - Kt/2.303$

8. In case of $K_a > K$, slope of extrapolated line is $-K/2.303$ and intercept is $(K_a F X_0)/[V_d(K_a - K)]$ ($\mu g/mL$) and slope of residual line is $-K_a/2.303$

9. Overall Elimination Rate Constant of Parent Drug $K(\,h^{-1}) = (-\text{Slope})$ X 2.303

10. Elimination Half – Life of parent drug $t_{1/2}$ (h) $= 0.693/K$

11. Absorption rate constant $K_a(\,h\,r^{-1}) = (-\text{Slope}) \times 2.303$

12. Absorption Half Life of drug $t_{\frac{1}{2}} = 0.693/ K_a$

13. Area Under the Plasma– Time Curve AUC_0^{∞} ($\mu g.h/mL$)= $AUC_0^{\,t} +$ $AUC_t^{\,\infty}$

    $AUC_0^{\,t}$ (Trapezoidal Rule) ($\mu g.h/mL$) = $[(C_0 + C_1)/2]\,(t_1 - t_0) + (C_1 + C_2)\,(t_2 - t_1)/2 + ----+ (C_{n-1} + C_n)\,(t_n - t_{n-1})/2$

    AUC_t^{∞} (Integration Method) ($\mu g.h/mL$) = C_{last} / K

14. Area Under the Mean Curve $AUMC_0^{\infty}$ ($\mu g.h^2/mL$) = $AUMC_0^{\,t} +$ $AUMC_t^{\infty}$

    $AUMC_0^{\,t}$ (Trapezoidal Rule) ($\mu g.h^2/mL$)

    $AUMC_t^{\infty}$ ($\mu g.h^2/mL$) = $C_{last}\, t_{last} /K + C_{last} / K^2$

15. Mean Residence Time (H) = $AUMC_0^{\infty}/ AUC_0^{\infty} = 1/K + 1/K_a$

16. Volume of Distribution V_d (L)= $K_a\, F\, X_0\, /$ Intercept $(K_a - K)$

17. Total clearance CL_T (L/h) = $V_d.K$ or FX_0 / AUC

18. $t_{max} = 2.303 \log (K_a/K) / (K_a{-}K)$

19. $C_{max} = (FX_0 . e_{-ktmax})/V$

20. Lag time $(t_0) = (\ln A - \ln B)/ (K_a{-}K)$ where A and B are intercept values of both   residual lines and extrapolated line

WAGNER NELSON METHOD

1. Wagner Nelson method is used alternatively for determination of Absorption Rate constant. The equation is given below.

$$\text{Log} [(A_\infty/V_d) - (A_t/V_d)] = \text{Log } C_0{-}K_a t/2.303$$

2. Graph on semilogarthmic paper by taking log percent unabsorbed $[(A_\infty/V_d) - (A_t/V_d)]$ on Y axis and time on X axis will givea a straight line with negative slope which is equivalent to absorption rate constant.

3. This method allows to understand the absorption kinetics without any prior assumption

4. This method is also useful for studying the mechanisms of drug release from dosage form *invivo*

5. It is direct method to determine absorption rate constant.

One Compartment Open Model – Extravascular – Urine – Parent Drug

Schematic Representation

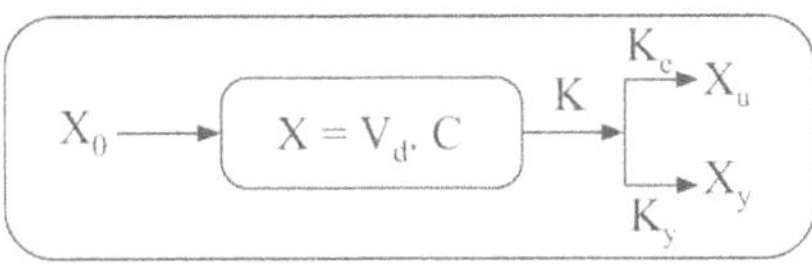

X_0 -   Dose Administered (mg)

X -   Amount of Drug present in the compartment at any time 't'

V_d -   Apparent Volume of distribution (mL or L)

C -   Plasma Concentration (μg/mL or ng/mL)

K -   Overall Apparent Elimination Rate Constant (h^{-1})

K_a -   First order absorption rate const (h^{-1})

K_e -   Excretion rate constant through renal pathway (h^{-1})

K_y -   Excretion rate constant through non renal pathway (h^{-1})

X_u - Cumulative Amount of drug that ultimately excreted through renal pathway

X_y - Cumulative Amount of drug that ultimately excreted t/h non renal pathway

EXCRETION RATE METHOD

Final Equation: $\text{Log}\ (\Delta X_u/\Delta t) = \text{Log}\ [(K_e K_a F X_0)/ (K_a-K)] - (Kt^1/2.303)$

Formulae

1. Intercept $= [(K_e K_a F X_0)/ (K_a-K)]$

2. Overall elimination rate constant (K) $=$ (–Slope of extrapolated line) $\times\ 2.303$

3. Absorption rate constant $(K_a) =$ (–Slope of residual line) $\times\ 2.303$

4. Excretion rate constant through renal pathway $(K_e) =$ (Intercept) $(K_a-K)/ K_a F X_0$

5. Elimination half life $= 0.693/K$

6. Absorption half life $= 0.693/K_a$

7. Excretion rate constant through non renal pathway $(k_y) = K-K_e$

8. Fraction of dose excreted through renal pathway $(f_e) = K_e/K$

SIGMA MINUS METHOD

Final Equation: $\text{Log}\ (X_u^{\infty}-X_u^t) = \text{Log}\ [(X_u^{\infty}.K_a) / (K_a-K)] - (K_t/2.303)$

$$X_u^{\infty} = K_e F X_0/K$$

Formulae

1. Intercept $= [(X_u^{\infty}.K_a) / (K_a-K)]$

2. Overall elimination rate constant (K) $=$ (–Slope of extrapolated line) $\times\ 2.303$

3. Absorption rate constant $(K_a) =$ (–Slope of residual line) $\times\ 2.303$

4. Excretion rate constant through renal pathway $(K_e) =$ (Intercept) $(K_a-K)/ K_a F X_0$

5. Elimination half life $= 0.693/K$

6. Absorption half life $= 0.693/K_a$

7. Excretion rate constant through non renal pathway $(k_y) = K-K_e$

8. Fraction of dose excreted through renal pathway $(f_e) = K_e/K$

Two Compartment Open Model – I.V
Bolus – Plasma – Parent Drug

Schematic Representation

$$X_0 \longrightarrow \boxed{X_c = V_c \cdot C} \underset{K_{21}}{\overset{K_{12}}{\rightleftarrows}} \boxed{X_2 = V_t \cdot C_t}$$
$$\downarrow K_{13}$$
$$X_3$$

X_0 — Dose Administered (mg)

X_c — Amount of Drug present in the central compartment at any time 't'

X_t — Amount of Drug present in the tissue compartment at any time 't'

X_3 — Amount of Drug eliminated from central compartment at any time 't'

V_c — Apparent Volume of distribution of central compartment (mL or L)

V_t — Apparent Volume of distribution of tissue compartment (mL or L)

C — Plasma Concentration (μg/mL or ng/mL)

C_t — Tissue concentration (μg/mL or ng/mL)

K_{12} — Micro constant for the distribution of drug from compartment 1 to 2 (h^{-1})

K_{21} — Micro constant for the distribution of drug from compartment 2 to 1 (h^{-1})

K_{13} — Overall Elimination Rate constant of drug from central compt. (h^{-1})

Final Equation

$$C = A\, e^{-\alpha t} + B\, e^{-\beta t}$$

Where $A = [X_0 (\alpha - K_{21})] / Vc\, (\alpha - \beta)$

$B = [X_0 (K_{21} - \beta)] / Vc\, (\alpha - \beta)$

Graph on Semi log Paper

X axis – Time (hours); Y axis – Plasma parent drug concentration (μg/mL)

1. Bi exponential curve will be obtained. By considering the last two points of straight curve extrapolate the curve on to Y- axis. This Line is called as **Extrapolated line**.

2. Now determine the Plasma concentrations on the extrapolated line at each time intervals. These concentrations are known as **Extrapolated Concentrations** which are denoted with **C***

3. Now substract the each plasma concentrations from extrapolated concentrations. These obtained concentrations are known as **Residual Concentrations.**

$$C_r = C^* - C$$

4. Now draw a line by pointing residual concentration values at each time period. This line is called as **Residual Line.**

Precautions to be taken while plotting the Graph

1. Y- Intercept of both extrapolated line and residual line should not be the same value. (when there is no lag time)
2. Draw a best fit residual line so that it should be greater than the Y-intercept of extrapolated line.
3. For the determination of slope of extrapolated line consider last two points only.
4. For the determination of slope of residual line any two points can be considered which are coming on residual line.

Formulae:

1. Intercept of Extrapolated line = B = $[X_0 (K_{21} - \beta)] / V_c (\alpha - \beta)$ (μg/mL)
2. Intercept of Residual line = A = $[X_0 (\alpha - K_{21})] / V_c (\alpha - \beta)$ (μg/mL)
3. Slope of extrapolated line = $[\log (C_2) - \log (C_1)] / (t_2 - t_1) = -\beta/2.303$
4. Slope of residual line = $[\log (C_2) - \log (C_1)] / (t_2 - t_1) = -\alpha/2.303$
5. Rate constant of extrapolated line (β) = $-$(slope of extrapolated line) $\times$ 2.303 (h^{-1})
6. Rate constant of residual line (α) = $-$(slope of residual line)$\times$ 2.303 (h^{-1})
7. Initial Plasma Concentration C_0 = A + B (μg/mL)
8. $K_{21} (h^{-1})$ = $(\alpha B + \beta A) / (A + B)$
9. $K_{10} (h^{-1})$ = $\alpha \beta / K_{21}$ (or) $[\alpha \beta(A+B)] / (\alpha B + \beta A)$
10. $K_{12} (h^{-1})$ = $\alpha + \beta - K_{21} - K_{10}$ (or) $[AB (\alpha - \beta)^2] / [(A+B)(\alpha B + \beta A)]$
11. Amount of the drug present in tissue compartment
$$(X_t) (mg) = (K_{12}X_0) (e^{-\beta t} - e^{-\alpha t}) / (\alpha - \beta)$$

12. t_{max} in tissue compartment $=[\ln(\alpha /\beta)]/(\alpha - \beta)$

13. Area Under the curve $= (A/\alpha) + (B/\beta)$

14. Volume of distribution of Central Compartment $(V_c) = X_0/(A + B)$ or X_0 / K_{10} AUC

15. Volume of distribution at steady state $(Vd_{ss}) = [(K_{12}+ K_{21})/K_{21}]\, V_c$

16. Volume of distribution of tissue compartment $(V_t) = Vd_{ss} - V_c$

17. Volume of distribution by area $(Vd_{area}) = K_{10}.V_c/\beta$ (or) $X_0 / $ AUC. B

18. Volume of distribution by extrapolation $(Vd_{exp}) = X_0/ B$
    (or) $[V_c (\alpha - \beta)] / (K_{21} - \beta)$

19. Clearance $= K_{10} \times V_c$ (or) $X_0 / $ AUC

20. $Vd_{exp} > Vd_{area} > Vd_{ss} > V_c$

TWO COMPARTMENT OPEN MODEL –EXTRAVASCULAR – PLASMA – PARENT DRUG

Schematic Representation:

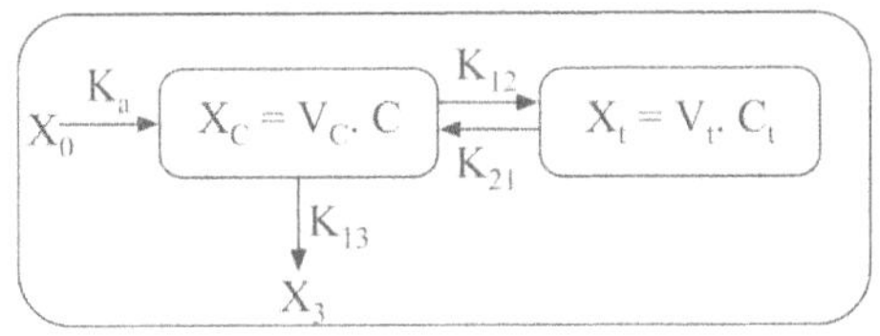

X_0	Dose Administered (mg)
X_c	Amount of Drug present in the central compartment at any time't'
X_t	Amount of Drug present in the tissue compartment at any time't'
X_3	Amount of Drug eliminated from central compartment at any time 't'
V_c	Apparent Volume of distribution of central compartment (mL or L)
V_t	Apparent Volume of distribution of tissue compartment (mL or L)
C	Plasma Concentration (µg/mL or ng/mL)
C_t	Tissue concentration (µg/mL or ng/mL)
K_{12}	Micro constant for the distribution of drug from compartment 1 to 2 (h^{-1})

K_{21} Micro constant for the distribution of drug from compartment 2 to 1 (h^{-1})

K_{13} Overall Elimination Rate constant of drug from central compt. (h^{-1})

Ka First order absorption rate constant (h^{-1})

Final Equation: $C = A\,e^{-\alpha t} + B\,e^{-\beta t} - C_0\,e^{-Kat}$

$$\text{Where } A = [FX_0\,(\alpha - K_{21})] \,/\, [V_c\,(\alpha - \beta)]$$

$$B = [FX_0\,(K_{21} - \beta)] \,/\, [V_c\,(\alpha - \beta)]$$

Graph on Semi log Paper:

X axis – Time (min / hours / days)

Y axis – Plasma parent drug concentration (μg/mL or ng/mL or mg/mL)

(a) Bi exponential curve will be obtained. By considering the last two points of straight curve extrapolate the curve on to Y- axis. This Line is called as **First Extrapolated line**. Now determine the Plasma concentrations on the extrapolated line at each time intervals. These concentrations are known as **First Extrapolated Concentrations** which are denoted with **C***. Now substract the each plasma concentrations from extrapolated concentrations. These obtained concentrations are known as **First Residual Concentrations**. $C_r = C^* - C$

(b) Now plot a graph by pointing first residual concentration values at each time period. Again bi exponential curve will be obtained. By considering the last two points of straight curve extrapolate the curve on to Y- axis. This Line is called as **Second Extrapolated line**. Now determine the Plasma concentrations on the extrapolated line at each time intervals. These concentrations are known as **Second Extrapolated Concentrations** which are denoted with **C****. Now substract the each plasma concentrations from extrapolated concentrations. These obtained concentrations are known as **Second Residual Concentrations**. $C_r = C^{**} - C$. Now draw a straight line (residual line) by pointing second residual concentration values at each time period.

Note: Total of three different Y- Intercept values should be obtained.

Formulae

1. C_0 = Y-intercept of residual line = A+B

2. A = Y-intercept of second extrapolated line

3. B = Y-intercept of first extrapolated line

4. α = (–Slope of second extrapolated line × 2.303)

5. β = (–Slope of first extrapolated line × 2.303)

6. Ka = (-Slope of residual line × 2.303)

7. $V_c = (FX_0) / [(A/\alpha) + (B/\beta) + (C_0/K_a)]$

8. $Cl = K_{10} V_c$

MULTIPLE DOSE INJECTIONS

Formulae

1. $R = e^{-kT}$ where T is the dosing interval

2. $C_{max} = C_1^0 / 1{-}R$

3. $C_{min} = R\, C_{max} = R\,(C_1^0 / 1{-}R)$

4. $C_{ave} = [AUC]_{t1}^{t2} / T = X_0 / (V_d K T)$

5. $X_{max} = X_0 / 1{-}R$

6. $X_{min} = R\, X_{max}$

7. $X_{ave} = X_0 / kT$

8. Plasma concentration at any time after n^{th} dose

    $C_n t = C_0 [(1- e^{-nkT}) / (1-e^{-kT})]\, e^{-kt}$

9. Plasma concentration at any time after achieving steady state level

    $C_n\infty = C_0 [1/ (1-e^{-kT})]\, e^{-kt}$

10. Loading Dose $X^* = C_{ave}\, Vd/ e^{-kT}$

11. Maintenance dose $= X^* (1{-}R)$

12. Accumulation Index $R_{ac} = 1/1{-}R$

MULTIPLE DOSE ORAL ADMINISTRATION

Formulae

(a) $R = e^{-kT}$ where T is the dosing interval

$$C_t^n = \frac{K_a F X_0}{V_d\left(K_a - K\right)}\left[\frac{1-e^{-nkT}}{1-e^{-kT}}e^{-kt} - \frac{1-e^{-nk_a T}}{1-e^{-k_a T}}e^{-K_a t}\right]$$

(b) Plasma concentration at any time after n^{th} dose

$$C_t^{\infty} = \frac{K_a F X_0}{V_d (K_a - K)} \left[\frac{e^{-kT}}{1 - e^{-kT}} - \frac{e^{-k_a T}}{1 - e^{-k_a T}} \right]$$

(c) Plasma concentration at any time after achieving steady state level.

(d) Maximum Plasma Concentration.

$$C_{max} = \frac{K_a F X_0}{V_d (K_a - K)} \left[\frac{e^{-K t_{max}}}{1 - e^{-kT}} - \frac{e^{-k_a t_{max}}}{1 - e^{-kaT}} \right]$$

$$C_{max} = \frac{K_a F X_0}{V_d (K_a - K)} \left[\frac{1}{1 - e^{-kT}} - \frac{1}{1 - e^{-k_a T}} \right]$$

(e) Minimum Plasma Concentration

(f) Average Plasma Concentration

$$C_{ave} = {}_{[}AUC]_{t1}{}^{t2} / T = F X_0 / (V_d K T)$$

(g) Loading Dose $X^* = (C_{ave} V_d / e^{-kT}) / F$

(h) Maintenance Dose $= X^* (1 - R)$

(i) Accumulation Index $R_{ac} = 1 / (1 - R)$

APPENDIX 9

BUFFERS AND REAGENTS

1. **Boric Acid and Potassium Chloride, 0.2 M:** Dissolve 12.366 g of boric acid and 14.911 g of potassium chloride in water and dilute with water to 1000 mL.

2. **Disodium Hydrogen Phosphate, 0.2 M:** Dissolve 71.630 g of disodium hydrogen phosphate in water and dilute with water to 1000 mL.

3. **Hydrochloric Acid, 0.2 M:** Hydrochloric acid diluted with water to contain 7.292 g of HCl in 1000 mL.

4. **Potassium Chloride, 0.2 M:** Dissolve 14.911 g of potassium chloride in water and dilute with water to 1000 mL.

5. **Potassium Dihydrogen Phosphate, 0.2 M:** Dissolve 27.218 g of potassium dihydrogen phosphate in water and dilute with water to 1000 mL.

6. **Potassium Hydrogen Phthalate, 0.2 M:** Dissolve 40.846 g of potassium hydrogen phthalate in water and dilute with water to 1000 mL.

7. **Sodium Hydroxide, 0.2 M:** Dissolve sodium hydroxide in water to produce a 40 to 60% w/v solution and allow standing. Taking precautions to avoid absorption of carbon dioxide, siphon off the clear supernatant liquid and dilute with carbon dioxide-free water a suitable volume of the liquid to contain 8.0 g of NaOH in 1000 mL.

   Note – 0.2 M Sodium hydroxide must not be used later than one month after preparation.

8. **Phosphate Buffer:** Place 50.0 mL of 0.2 M potassium dihydrogen phosphate in a 200-mL volumetric flask, add the specified volume of 0.2 M sodium hydroxide (see Table) and then add water to volume.

Table

pH	0.2MNaOH, mL	pH	0.2MNaOH, mL
5.8	3.6	7.0	29.1
6.0	5.6	7.2	34.7
6.2	8.1	7.4	39.1
6.4	11.6	7.6	42.4
6.6	16.4	7.8	44.5
6.8	22.4	8.0	46.1

9. **Acetate Buffer pH 2.8:** Dissolve 4 g of anhydrous sodium acetate in about 840 mL of water, add sufficient glacial acetic acid to adjust the pH to 2.8 (about 155 mL) and dilute with water to 1000 mL.

10. **Acetate Buffer pH 3.4:** Mix 50 mL of 0.1M sodium acetate with 950 mL of 0.1M acetic acid.

11. **Acetate Buffer pH 3.5:** Dissolve 25 g of ammonium acetate in 25 mL of water and add 38 mL of 7M hydrochloric acid. Adjust the pH to 3.5 with either 2M hydrochloric acid or 6M ammonia and dilute with water to 100 mL.

12. **Acetate Buffer pH 3.7:** Dissolve 10 g of anhydrous sodium acetate in 300 mL of water, adjust to pH to 3.7 with glacial acetic acid and dilute with water to 1000 mL. Before use adjust to pH 3.7, if necessary, with glacial acetic acid or anhydrous sodium acetate, as required.

13. **Acetate Buffer pH 4.0:** Place 2.86 mL of glacial acetic acid and 1.0 mL of a 50% w/v solution of sodium hydroxide in a 100-mL volumetric flask, add water to volume and mix. Adjust the pH, if necessary.

14. **Acetate Buffer pH 4.4:** Dissolve 136 g of sodium acetate and 77 g of ammonium acetate in water and dilute with water to 1000 mL. Add 250 mL of glacial acetic acid and mix

15. **Acetate Buffer pH 4.6:** Dissolve 5.4 g of sodium acetate in 50 mL of water, add 2.4 mL of glacial acetic acid and dilute with water to 100 mL. Adjust the pH, if necessary.

16. **Acetate Buffer pH 4.7:** Dissolve 8.4 g of sodium acetate and 3.35 mL of glacial acetic acid in sufficient water to produce 1000 mL. Adjust the pH, if necessary.

17. **Acetate Buffer pH 5.0:** Dissolve 13.6 g of sodium acetate and 6 mL of glacial acetic acid in sufficient water to produce 1000 mL. Adjust the pH, if necessary.

18. **Acetate Buffer pH 5.5:** Dissolve 272 g of sodium acetate in 500 mL of water by heating to 35°, cool and add slowly 50 mL of glacial acetic acid and sufficient water to produce 1000 mL. Adjust the pH, if necessary.

19. **Acetate Buffer pH 6.0:** Dissolve 100 g of ammonium acetate in 300 mL of water, add 4.1 mL of glacial acetic acid, adjust the pH, if necessary, using 10M ammonia or 5M acetic acid and dilute with water to 500 mL.

20. **Phosphate Buffer pH 2.0:** Dissolve 0.136 g of potassium dihydrogen phosphate in 800 mL of water, adjust the pH to 2.0 with hydrochloric acid and add sufficient water to produce 1000 mL.

21. **Phosphate Buffer pH 2.5:** Dissolve 100 g of potassium dihydrogen phosphate in 800 mL of water, adjust the pH to 2.5 with hydrochloric acid and add sufficient water to produce 1000 mL.

22. **Phosphate Buffer pH 3.6:** Dissolve 0.900 g of anhydrous disodium hydrogen phosphate and 1.298 g of citric acid monohydrate in sufficient water to produce 1000 mL.

23. **Phosphate Buffer pH 4.0, Mixed:** Dissolve 5.04 g disodium hydrogen phosphate and 3.01 g of potassium dihydrogen phosphate in sufficient water to produce 1000 mL. Adjust the pH with glacial acetic acid.

24. **Phosphate Buffer pH 4.9:** Dissolve 40 g of sodium dihydrogen phosphate and 1.2 g of sodium hydroxide in sufficient water to produce 100 mL. If necessary, adjust the pH with 1M sulphuric acid or 1M sodium hydroxide as required.

25. **Phosphate Buffer pH 5.0:** Dissolve 6.8 g of potassium dihydrogen phosphate in 1000 mL of water and adjust the pH to 5.0 with 10M potassium hydroxide.

26. **Simulated Gastric Fluid (SGF):** Dissolve 2.0 g of sodium chloride and 3.2 g of purified pepsin that is derived from porcine stomach mucosa, with an activity of 800 to 2500 units per mg of protein, in 7.0 mL of hydrochloric acid and sufficient water to make 1000 mL. This test solution has a pH of about 1.2

27. **Simulated Intestinal Fluid (SIF):** Dissolve 6.8 g of monobasic potassium phosphate in 250 mL of water, mix, and add 77 mL of 0.2 N sodium hydroxide and 500 mL of water. Add 10.0 g of pancreatin, mix, and adjust the resulting solution with either 0.2 N sodium hydroxide or 0.2 N hydrochloric acid to a pH of 6.8 ± 0.1. Dilute with water to 1000 mL

28. **Hydrochloric Acid (0.1 N):** Dilute 8.5 mL of concentrated hydrochloric acid to 1000 mL.

29. **Sodium Hydroxide (0.1 N):** Dissolve 4 g of NaoH in 1000 mL of distilled water.

APPENDIX 10

VIVA-VOCE QUESTIONS

1. Salicylic acid reacts with Fecl$_3$ to give violet color. Give the reason.

2. What is the range of visible region?

3. What is the source of light in colorimeter?

4. What is the range of visible region?

5. What is the source of light and detector used in UV spectrophotometer?

6. Define Compartment.

7. What is open model?

8. Mention different Pharmacokinetic models.

9. Define Zero order and First order kinetics with examples.

10. Define Linear and Non-linear kinetics and give examples.

11. Define the following

    (a) AUC and its significance

    (b) Half-life and its significance

    (c) Apparent Volume of distribution and its significance

    (d) Clearance and its significance

12. Define Bioavailability.

13. Define Absorption.

14. Define Absolute and Relative bioavailability.

15. Compare and Contrast Excretion rate and Sigma-minus method.

16. What are the assumptions in deriving first order equation in one compartment open model?

17. What is Organ Clearance?

18. What is Renal Clearance?

19. What is Hepatic clearance?

20. What is Therapeutic Index?

21. Define Renal clearance ratio.

22. Define Renal function.

23. Define the following

   (a) Bio-pharmaceutics

   (b) Pharmacokinetics

   (c) Clinical Pharmacokinetics

   (d) Chrono-pharmacokinetics

   (e) Bioequivalence

24. Define distribution.

25. What is protein binding?

26. What is Displacement interaction? Give classical example.

27. Give the classical example for Food-Drug interaction.

28. What are different methods to study Protein binding?

29. What is Dialysis?

30. What is Scatchard Plot?

31. What is the significance of Scatchard plot?

32. What is Lineweaver-Burk plot?

33. Write the inter relationship between $t_{1/2}$, V_d and Clearance?

34. What is Synergism and give classical example.

35. What is Dissolution rate?

36. Mention dissolution apparatus official in I.P.

37. What is *in vitro in vivo* correlation?

38. Define Noyes Whitney equation.

39. Define Henderson hasselbach equations for weak acid and weak base.

40. Define Fick's law of diffusion.

41. What is Sink condition?

42. Mention different approaches to maintain Sink condition.

43. What is Passive diffusion?

44. What is Active transport?

45. Define Sustained release formulation.

46. List out the techniques to design SR.

47. Mention the examples of polymers used in SR.

48. What are the advantages of SR.?

49. Differentiate SR and Controlled release.

50. Mention the limitations of SR.

51. What is Maintenance dose?

52. What is Loading dose?

53. Mention the Pharmacokinetic parameters on which Loading dose is dependent.

54. Mention the Pharmacokinetic parameters on which Maintenance dose is dependent.

55. What is an Ointment? Mention different Ointment bases with examples.

56. Define Solubility?

57. Mention different approaches of Solubilization.

58. Mention different mechanisms of dissolution.

59. List out the official tests for tablets in I.P.

60. Mention the Acceptance criteria for dissolution of tablets in I.P.

61. Mention the Acceptance criteria for dissolution of enteric coated tablets in I.P.

62. What is enteric coating? Give classes of drugs which require enteric coating.

63. Give examples of polymers used in Enteric coating.

64. What is Pinocytosis?

65. Define Biotransformation.

66. Mention different Phase II reactions.

67. What is entero-hepatic circulation?

68. What is first pass effect? Mention different ways to overcome this?
69. How micronization increases the dissolution of drugs?
70. What is polymorphism?
71. What are the advantages of buffered aspirin tablets?
72. Give examples for the drugs which cause enzyme induction.
73. Give examples for the drugs which cause enzyme inhibition.
74. Define prodrug.
75. What is Glomerular filtration rate? How it is determined?
76. Give examples of drugs which undergo Enterohepatic circulation.
77. Give the significance of Enterohepatic circulation.
78. Define MRT.
79. What is Therapeutic Drug Monitoring?
80. Give classes of drugs which require TDM.
81. What is the importance of Glutathione conjugation?
82. Give the metabolic reactions for paracetamol.
83. What is Gastric emptying?
84. Give the descending order of the formulations with respect to their bioavailability.
85. What are the limitations of pH partition hypothesis?
86. How salt form of a drug improves the solubility?
87. What is solid dispersion?
88. What is Hixson – Crowell's cube root law of dissolution?
89. Give examples of drugs which require carrier mediated transport.
90. What is Paracellular transport?
91. What is Transcellular transport?
92. Explain a typical plasma concentration - time profile following oral administration.
93. What is Latin square cross over design?
94. What is the difference between Serum and Plasma?
95. What is student't' test?

96. How slope is calculated?

97. How slope is calculated statistically?

98. What is Correlation coefficient?

99. What is Regression analysis?

100. What is ANOVA?

101. What is Michaelis menton kinetics?

www.ingramcontent.com/pod-product-compliance
Lightning Source LLC
LaVergne TN
LVHW011923160726
843514LV00004B/897